SEXUAL PROBLEMS OF ADOLESCENTS IN INSTITUTIONS

SEXUAL PROBLEMS OF ADOLESCENTS IN INSTITUTIONS

Edited by

DAVID A. SHORE, M.S.W.

*Program Manager, Quality Assurance in Psychiatry
and Substance Abuse
Joint Commission on Accreditation of Hospitals
Founding Editor, Journal of Social Work & Human Sexuality
Editor, Human Sexuality Update*

and

HARVEY L. GOCHROS

*University of Hawaii at Manoa
School of Social Work
Director, Social Work Program for the Study of Sex
University of Hawaii*

With a Foreword by

William A. Granzig, Ph.D.

*Executive Director
American Association of Sex Educators,
Counselors, and Therapists*

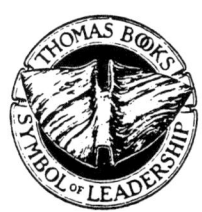

CHARLES C THOMAS • PUBLISHER
Springfield • Illinois • U.S.A.

Published and Distributed Throughout the World by
CHARLES C THOMAS • PUBLISHER
Bannerstone House
301-327 East Lawrence Avenue, Springfield, Illinois, U.S.A.

This book is protected by copyright. No part of it
may be reproduced in any manner without written
permission from the publisher.

© *1981, by* CHARLES C THOMAS • PUBLISHER
ISBN 0-398-04143-1 (cloth)
ISBN 0-398-04144-X (paper)
Library of Congress Catalog Card Number: 80-20772

With THOMAS BOOKS careful attention is given to all details of manufacturing and design. It is the Publisher's desire to present books that are satisfactory as to their physical qualities and artistic possibilities and appropriate for their particular use. THOMAS BOOKS will be true to those laws of quality that assure a good name and good will.

Printed in the United States of America
I-R X-1

Library of Congress Cataloging in Publication Data

Main entry under title:

Sexual problems of adolescents in institutions.

Includes bibliographies and index.
 1. Youth--Sexual behavior--Addresses, essays, lectures. 2. Sex instruction--Addresses, essays, lectures. 3. Children--Institutional care--United States--Addresses, essays, lectures. I. Shore, David A. II. Gochros, Harvey L.
HQ27.S49   362.7'96   80-20772
ISBN 0-398-04143-1
ISBN 0-398-04144-X (pbk.)

CONTRIBUTORS

Jack S. Annon, Ph.D. Graduate Affiliate Faculty, Department of Psychology; Associate Clinical Professor, Department of Psychiatry, University of Hawaii; Senior Consultant for Sexual Counseling Services, Department of Obstetrics and Gynecology.

Miranda S. Arnow, B.S.W. Medical Social Worker, Summit Medical Center, Milwaukee, Wisconsin; Sexual Assault Treatment Center, Family Hospital.

Diane Blake Brashear, Ph.D. President, Brashear Center, Indianapolis, Indiana; Lecturer, School of Social Work, Indiana University.

Donald D. Brown, Ph.D. Associate Professor, Department of Health Education, Trenton State College, Trenton, New Jersey.

Linda Carelli, M.S.W. Assistant Professor, Graduate School of Social Work, Rutgers University, New Brunswick, New Jersey; Former staff member, Willowbrook State School.

Joel Fischer, D.S.W. Professor, School of Social Work, University of Hawaii.

Randal G. Forrester. Executive Director, Persad Center, Inc., Pittsburgh, Pennsylvania.

Charles A. Glisson, Ph.D. Associate Professor, School of Social Work, University of Hawaii; Former ward director, Bryce State Hospital, Tuscaloosa, Alabama.

Jean S. Gochros, D.S.W. Candidate, School of Social Work, University of Denver, Denver, Colorado; Private practice.

Erwin J. Haeberle, Ph.D. Director of Historical Research, Institute for Advanced Study of Human Sexuality, San Francisco, California.

David A. Iacono-Harris, Ph. D. Assistant Professor and Director of Social Work Program, Department of Sociology and Social Work, Elizabethtown College, Elizabethtown, Pennsylvania.

Delene Iacono-Harris, M.S.S.W. Instructor, Department of Sociology and Social Work, Elizabethtown College, Elizabethtown, Pennsylvania.

James Huggins, M.S.W. Director of Programing, Persad Center, Inc., Pittsburgh, Pennsylvania.

Joy D. Johnson, M.A. Associate Professor, Jane Addams College of Social Work, University of Illinois at Chicago Circle, Chicago, Illinois; Former service chief of adolescent unit, Department of Mental Health, Chicago, Illinois.

Burton Joseph, J.D. Chairperson, Board of Directors, The Playboy Foundation, Chicago, Illinois; Faculty, Illinois Institute of Technology, Chicago Kent College of Law, Chicago, Illinois; Member, Board of Directors, American Civil Liberties Union; Member Chicago Bar Association Commission on Juvenile and Adolescent Offenders.

Winifred Kempton, M.S.S. Consultant for education and training, Planned Parenthood of Southeastern Pennsylvania; Trainer in private practice on sexuality and disability.

O. Dale Kunkel, D.S.W. Assistant Professor, School of Social Work, University of Oklahoma, Norman, Oklahoma; Former interim clinical director, Teenage Resource Center, Fullerton, California.

Larry Lister, D.S.W. Associate Professor and Coordinator of Continuing Education, School of Social Work, University of Hawaii, Honolulu, Hawaii; Former Director of Social Services, Leahi Hospital, Honolulu, Hawaii.

Ord Matek, M.A. Associate Professor, Jane Addams College of Social Work, University of Illinois at Chicago Circle, Chicago, Illinois; Faculty member, Illinois School of Professional Psychology, Chicago, Illinois: Former director of residential treatment program for seriously emotionally disturbed adolescents.

Gerald J. Murphy, D.S.W. Consultant, Madonna Manor/Hope Haven Home for Boys, New Orleans, Louisiana; Former priest.

Craig H. Robinson, Ph.D. Assistant Clinical Professor, Department of Psychology, University of Hawaii, Honolulu, Hawaii Private practice in clinical psychology.

LeRoy G. Schultz, M.S.W. Professor, School of Social Work, West Virginia University, Morgantown, West Virginia.

Margaret Standish. Executive Director, The Playboy Foundation, Chicago, Illinois.

TO

Ruth and Milton Shore for all their love, and to Jeffrey Shore and Gloria Graff for always being there.

and

To Jean Schaar Gochros for her understanding and help on matters both professional and personal, and to Susan and David Gochros, who have reminded me of the problems, opportunities and joys of adolescence.

FOREWORD

IN the midst of our society's growing preoccupation and openness about sexuality, certain populations have been somehow overlooked. American Association of Sex Educators, Counselors and Therapists, itself, is becoming more and more concerned with such previously ignored groups.

Institutionalized adolescents are among these sexually ignored groups, despite the fact that they are often at the peak of their sexual energy, curiosity, and activity. Their normal adolescent sexual needs and concerns are often both aggravated and exagerated by the fact that they are living in close contact with many other adolescents. Yet, often their natural urges for sexual expression are surpressed and any overt expression of their sexuality may be considered undesirable or even pathological by those responsible for their care. With the *Sexual Problems of Adolescents in Institutions,* David Shore and Harvey Gochros have brought this subject out of the silence which has too long surrounded it.

This book of original contributions proceeds in an orderly fashion from describing the nature and origin of the sexual oppression of both adolescents and the institutionalized in general, and institutionalized adolescents in particular. It then proceeds to describe the particular problems of each of the diverse types of settings in which adolescents reside. Moreover, it rationally explores the problems inherent in determining how best to meet the sexual needs of adolescents in residential facilities consistent with the divergent pressures which influence their management such as legal matters, ethical issues, and administrative constraints.

Throughout, the book provides down-to-earth approaches to dealing with the complex problems inevitably encountered when adolescents must live in congregate living arrangements, without the security, individualized direction, sense of belonging and love that well functioning families can provide. For many adolescents, institutional care for varying lengths of time is the substitute for this type of family life.

Part of institutional care *must* be directed toward understanding and meeting the healthy sexual needs of adolescents as well as helping them develop into sexually functional and responsible adults. This book can assist concerned institutional staff and administrators in their day to day efforts to deal with the sexuality of their adolescents.

William A. Granzig

INTRODUCTION

IT has been estimated that more than one million American adolescents live, usually for reasons beyond their control, in institutions for the retarded, delinquent, emotionally disturbed, handicapped or chronically ill. [1] Many of these people are at the peak of their sexual energy, curiosity and activity. Yet, their sexual options are severely limited purely because they must live in institutions. The majority live in publicly supported residences in which overworked, underprepared staff are more concerned with maintaining order and following sex-negative institutional policies than they are with helping their residents develop functional and satisfying patterns of sexual expression. Adolescents in institutions encounter not only those problems commonly experienced by *any* adolescent, but the additional problems imposed on them by being confined to a long-term congregate care program.

Special Problems of Institutionalized Adolescents

Prisons often serve as the prototype of institutions. What is prison-like about prisons is found in varying degrees in institutions whose members have broken no law. More than seven times the number of institutionalized are confined, not for any wrongdoing, but because society believes it is for their own best interests. Whether confinement is intended to be benevolent or punitive, institutions resemble each other in their treatment of their residents. [2] Moreover, it is frequently suggested that institutional experiences are so similar because the pragmatic realities under which institutional staff and administrators must operate is so similar. As there are dramatic similarities in the treatment of institutional residents, it follows that the impact of institutionalization, particularly with regard to children and adolescents would have a more or less similar effect.

One study conducted at a long-term residential facility for physically handicapped children in Toronto determined the effects of institutionalization to be profound, long-lasting and damaging to the individual's ability to adjust to the outside world. As one of the few studies to address the sexual component, it found sexual counseling to be missing from the program, despite the fact that all patients interviewed expressed a desire to make potentially sexual contact with individuals who were not patients nor staff at the hospital.[3]

It is difficult to determine how best to meet the sexual needs of adolescents consistent with the divergent pressures which influence their management, such as legal, religious and ethical constraints. There are also the often more subtle influences of community attitudes and values — often quite sex-negative — which affect the ethos of institutions within a community.

Yet, despite such pressures, it is important for institutional staff to acknowledge the sexual needs and problems of adolescents in their institutions and to develop effective clinical, educational and management strategies to facilitate sexual development and expression in socially acceptable yet personally growth-producing ways. While institutional programs should draw from what we already know about adolescent sexuality, as well as from the numerous sex education programs now operating, each institution must take into account the unique circumstances and problems created by life in a long-term residential facility. Indeed the realities of residential living magnify the already complex tasks adolescents encounter as they negotiate this stage of sexual development.

In our sex-conscious age, it is becoming increasingly difficult for institutional staff and administrators to wear sexual blinders or try to "stamp out" sexual behavior in their institutions. It simply does not work. Rather, sexual behavior may manifest itself in less acceptable, more hidden and sometimes more violent ways. Once institutions accept the fact that the sexuality of their residents cannot be ignored, they will be in a better position to confront these issues directly. Such a direct approach will, as it has in

Introduction

the past, meet with considerable resistance from certain factions which believe that ignorance is bliss when it comes to sexuality. This belief usually is expressed as, "they (adolescents) don't know a damn thing about sex now and look at all the problems it creates! Can you imagine what would happen if we were to be more approving or even accepting of our residents' sexual expression?" This ignorance-is-more-blissful theory is not surprising. The notion that sexual education and "permissiveness" breeds sexual experimentation is a popular one. The evidence, however, does not support these concerns. Rather the data would suggest that responsible sex education and sexual counseling lead to more responsible sexual decision-making.

Educational and counseling programs should not be intended to extinguish sexual activity, nor should they focus exclusively on such critical concerns as the incidence of unwanted and unplanned pregnancies, sexually transmitted diseases and sexual victimology. However, such behaviors and their potential consequences are of great concern for all adolescents. They are particularly unacceptable in institutional settings in which the adolescent is often maintained at the state's expense, with the institution serving as substitute parents and without the support systems potentially available to adolescents living in their own homes. But beyond this content, in their role *in loco parentis* institutions must help those for whose care they are charged develop a positive sexual self image and begin to develop an approach to their sexual needs which will help them develop as happy, fulfilled and responsible human beings.

Purpose of This Book

The parameters of sexual problems of adolescents in institutions warrent a multifaceted approach. These various paths are explored in this book. The diversity of opinion to be found in these pages as well as the treatment, education and policy approaches are offered by the editors as the current state of the art. We recognize, however, that it is a very imperfect art. There are few areas of human life that are as subjective and thus, as controversial as human sexuality. We also realize the pressures, constraints and conflicting influences on institutional policy. For that reason, the editors have selected contributors for this book who are not only expert in the problems of adolescent sexuality, but are also conversant with the problems of institutional life.

Each of these authors recognizes the problems in determining how best to meet the sexual needs and regulate the sexual expression of adolescents in institutions consistent with the divergent pressures under which institutions exist. With this awareness, this book explores the sexual problems and needs of adolescents in diverse institutional settings, and suggests effective and humane clinical, educational and administrative interventions to facilitate functional sexual development and expression.

Organization of the Book

The book is organized in four major sections:

Section I: Historical and Social Perspectives includes three chapters which offer a perspective on the complexities of adult reactions to adolescent sexuality. The first chapter traces attitudes toward young people's sexual expression in those Western societies which have influenced our contemporary approach toward adolescent sexuality. Next there is an exploration of our contemporary attitudes and expectations about adolescent sexuality as well as the range of its expression. The section concludes with a discussion of the ethical and moral issues with which professional and lay people alike are currently struggling.

Section II: Management of Sexual Behavior includes five chapters which consider problems in institutional management of adolescent sexuality. A chapter on administrative concerns is followed by a review of legal issues which may influence administrative policy. The next two chapters suggest models for educational programs within institutions; one for residents, and the other for staff. The final chapter discusses the sensitive problem of sexual contact between institutional staff and residents.

Section III: Clinical Approaches focuses on treatment of sex-related problems within the institution. The section begins with a practical guide for handling day-to-day sex-related problems commonly encountered by institutional residents and staff. The next chapter presents a variety of approaches for changing dysfunctional sexual behavior of residents. A chapter on the use of group approaches for dealing with sexual problems and issues follows. The section concludes with an exploration of one of the most common areas of concern within institutions: homosexual behavior.

Section IV: Special Populations offers five chapters which describe the specific needs and problems of each of the most common populations served in institutions for adolescents: the dependent and neglected, the adjudicated delinquent, the emotionally disturbed, the mentally handicapped and, finally, the chronically ill and disabled.

The editors and contributors hope that this book will provide institutional staff with ideas for dealing with complex sex-related issues and the encouragement to do something more about them.

D. A. Shore
H. L. Gochros

Bibliography

1. Shore, D.A., *Sex in Institutions: A Review of the Literature,* Chicago: The Playboy Foundation, 1981.
2. Neier, A., "Sex and Confinement," *The Civil Liberties Review,* Vol. 5, No. 1, 1978, p. 6.
3. Carter, C., de Demeter, D., Fields, L., Jefferies, A. and Warren W., "The Impact of Institutionalization," *Dimensions of Health Services,* December, 1974, p. 43.

ACKNOWLEDGMENTS

WITH an original volume such as this, we wish to first and foremost thank our contributors. We deeply appreciate their willingness to tailor their experience, knowledge and insight for this present text.

We also wish to thank Jean Scharr Gochros and Ord Matek for their help and suggestions in this project.

Finally, to our publisher, Payne Thomas, for saintly patience and a most refreshing personal touch.

CONTENTS

Page

Foreword xi
Introduction xiii

Chapter

Part I
Historic and Social Perspectives

1. YOUTH AND SEX IN MODERN WESTERN SOCIETIES:
   A Historical Introduction
       Erwin J. Haeberle 3
2. CONTEMPORARY PATTERNS:
   Emerging Issues of the Sexual Rights of Adolescents in Institutions
       Diane Blake Brashear 17
3. THE INSTITUTIONALIZED ADOLESCENT
   AND THE ETHICS OF DESEXUALIZATION
       Gerald J. Murphy 27

Part II
Management of Sexual Behavior

4. ADMINISTRATIVE CONCERNS
       Ord Matek 36
5. LEGAL ISSUES
       Burton Joseph and Margaret Standish 51

6. SEX EDUCATION PROGRAMS FOR RESIDENTS
   Jean Schaar Gochros 56
7. IN-SERVICE TRAINING PROGRAMS FOR STAFF
   O. Dale Kunkel 71
8. SEXUAL CONTACT BETWEEN STAFF AND RESIDENTS
   LeRoy G. Schultz 90

Part III
Clinical Approaches

9. A PRACTICAL APPROACH TO DAY TO DAY
   SEXUAL PROBLEMS
   Jack S. Annon and Craig H. Robinson 104
10. CHANGING DYSFUNCTIONAL SEXUAL BEHAVIOR
    Joel Fischer and Miranda S. Arnow 118
11. INSTITUTIONAL GROUPS AND HUMAN SEXUALITY:
    Threatening or Therapeutic?
    Joy D. Johnson 139
12. HOMOSEXUALITY AND HOMOSEXUAL BEHAVIOR
    Randal G. Forrester and James Huggins 154

Part IV
Special Populations

13. SEX IN AN INSTITUTION FOR NEGLECTED
    AND DEPENDENT CHILDREN:
    A Personal Account
    Donald D. Brown 167
14. CORRECTIONAL FACILITIES
    Charles A. Glisson 180
15. EMOTIONALLY DISTURBED
    Delene Iacono-Harris and David A. Iacono-Harris 200
16. MENTALLY HANDICAPPED
    Winifred Kempton and Linda Carelli 210
17. CHRONICALLY ILL AND DISABLED
    Larry Lister 223

Index 237

SEXUAL PROBLEMS OF ADOLESCENTS IN INSTITUTIONS

PART I
HISTORIC AND SOCIAL PERSPECTIVES

Chapter One

YOUTH AND SEX IN MODERN WESTERN SOCIETIES:
A Historical Introduction

ERWIN J. HAEBERLE

IN the early seventeenth century, the French court physician Héroart kept a diary describing the education of the young dauphin, the future King Louis XIII. According to this detailed account, the infant prince had his penis frequently rubbed and caressed by his nurse and ladies of the court. As soon as he was able to walk about, he also became used to showing himself to adults, who would play with his penis and kiss it. Between the ages of four and six he was encouraged to go to bed with a number of nurses and ladies-in-waiting and to explore their vaginas. He also joined them when they had sexual intercourse with their husbands and even participated to some extent, for example by whipping their buttocks. Thus, he knew from personal observation how children are made, a lesson that was reinforced when his own father, King Henri IV, showed him the bed in which he had been conceived and then exposed himself to the boy, "stretching out his penis with his hand saying 'Behold what made you what you are.'"

Curiously enough, after the age of seven the prince was given to understand that the period of indiscriminate sex play was over and that he was expected to behave responsibly as an adult. He was dressed in adult clothes, with cloak and sword, and found himself more restricted. However, these new restrictions hardly amounted to sexual repression, because we find his Master of the Robe reporting to have met the dauphin once emerging from a bath with an erection. The alert attendant thereupon promptly proceeded to masturbate the adolescent with his hand — "a remedy which I have seen applied in England."[1]

Today, such child-rearing practices are certain to be condemned by most 'civilized' people, who may see in them nothing more than proof of the perversity and ignorance of a corrupt royal court. Furthermore, they may congratulate themselves on the educational progress that has made such conduct inconceivable for all classes of society — even aristocrats. However, if indeed one is right in calling this development progress, it can only be said to have taken a very peculiar route. Seen from our present standpoint, it seems at first to have been a regression to another extreme. For example, in the eighteenth century the French and English remedy for masturbation turned into a major cause of mental and physical illness. First an anonymous English pamphlet (*Onania or the Heinous Sin of Self-Pollution, and All its Frightful Consequences in both Sexes Considered,* 1710) and then a treatise in French, written by the Swiss Dr. Samuel Tissot (*L' Onanisme: Dissertation sur les Maladies produites par la Masturbation,* 1760) succeeded in convincing the European public that masturbation was a serious threat to human survival and that drastic steps had to be taken. Thus, by 1787, we find the German educators Oest and Campe winning a pedagogical prize with an essay that proposed a *Complete System for the Prevention of Self-Abuse.* With Teutonic thoroughness, they elaborate the following twenty theses:

> 1. One needs to emphasize the physical education, especially the physical toughening of children. 2. One needs to protect the young from solitude and leisure. 3. One must not make them tired or bored with their work. 4. One should protect the young from temptation. 5. One should not let them go to sleep too early or get up too late, lest they lie in bed awake. 6. One needs to ban thick and warm blankets. 7. One needs to prevent boys from putting their hands into the pockets of their trousers. 8. One needs to prevent girls from crossing their legs. 9. One needs to prevent two children from sleeping in the same bed. 10. One needs to prevent

any situation in which a rubbing of the sex organs is possible. 11. One needs to prevent several children, whether of different or the same sex, from ever being alone together. 12. One needs to impress the rules of modesty upon the young as early as possible. 13. One needs to protect the young from all sights that might harm their imagination. 14. One must take care to keep the food of the young simple, without too many spices. Neither should they be given warm or alcoholic drinks. 15. Children should take a daily bath in the summer and wash their secret parts with cold water in the winter. 16. One should not give children any premature social and literary education. 17. The few books which are suitable for children must be chosen with care. One must censor not only seductive passages, but also those that stimulate the imagination and arouse strong feelings in general. 18. One must prevent children from playing games such as "wedding" or "keeping house." 19. One must train children from the very beginning not to sleep lying on their backs, but only on their sides. 20. One must warn children as early as possible about the horrible consequences of abusing the organs of generation."[2]

Again, many modern readers may be disturbed by such educational principles and dismiss them as paranoid and totalitarian or, at best, as isolated examples of misguided zeal. However, just as in the earlier French medical diary, the German pedagocial essay reveals more than the personal idiosyncrasies of certain individuals, groups, or classes. Instead, both documents reflect vast social changes that transformed not only the external living conditions in the Western world but also the internal life, the psychology, the consciousness of the Western civilization. Certainly, the contrasts are striking. Our two sources reveal that within less than 200 years, a whole new concept of youthful development had taken hold. Not only had masturbation changed from therapy to disease, but the active encouragement of childhood sex play had turned into its absolute prohibition, and the simple early conferral of adult status on children had been replaced by an elaborate system of delaying social and intellectual maturity. As the prizewinning educators make quite clear, this system included the deliberate and prolonged infantilization of the young as well as their constant supervision and control. It alienated them from the natural responses of their own bodies and stifled their curiosity. Most important of all, it kept them dependent and thus not only extended the period of childhood but created an entirely new, protected period of life — adolescence.

It is important to realize, however, that the pedagogical crusade against masturbation, as indeed the whole sexual component of this increased repression, was not so much a cause as a symptom of the larger sociopsychological transformation mentioned above. This profound if gradual change, which is not easily explained and which escapes the static, ahistorical categories of orthodox sociology as practiced in the United States, was first analyzed and described by Norbert Elias as *The Civilizing Process* (1939).[3]

By examining and interpreting various literary sources from the Middle Ages to the Age of Enlightenment (mostly educational tracts and books of etiquette), Elias was able to demonstrate a considerable change in manners, which mirrored a corresponding change in sensibility. An ever-tightening self-discipline inhibited aggressive impulses and led to a growing revulsion toward the natural bodily functions. In fact, beginning in the seventeenth century, expert advice on proper eating and drinking, spitting, farting, urinating, defecating, blowing one's nose, washing, undressing, etc. can be observed becoming less and less explicit and, at the same time, more and more restrictive.

Elias documents that in the Middle Ages people blew their noses simply into their hands without regard for others until, in the thirteenth century, certain authorities on table manners demanded some refinement: "When you blow your nose. . ., turn round so that nothing falls on the table." Only much later, during the Renaissance, did the nobility begin to use handkerchiefs, but they remained rare and conspicuous signs of wealth. Even King Henri IV, the father of Louis XIII, owned only five handkerchiefs. The first monarch to have an abundant supply of them and to promote their general use, at least at court, was Louis XIV. The rules for blowing one's nose became more detailed and refined until, at the end of the eighteenth century, they again appeared terse and cryptic. One senses that the authors were growing uncomfortable with the subject and that they could already assume their readers to have a great deal of knowledge about the correct behavior. Apparently, several decades later all proper discretion could be taken for granted, because then the problem disappeared altogether from the literature.

Youth and Sex in Modern Western Societies

The preceding example is typical of changing Western attitudes with regard to all other bodily functions, including the sexual ones. As Western societies became more civilized, they became less spontaneous, more inhibited, disciplined, self-conscious, and self-controlled; in short, more adult. Behavior that once was perfectly acceptable in grown men and women was eventually tolerated only in children and finally extinguished even in them. Thus, our own children and adolescents have become both more innocent and more responsible than most of our ancestors ever were. Conversely, the adult of former centuries, if they could suddenly come to life, would strike us today as childish in their impulsiveness. Their lack of refinement and modesty, their impatience, their sudden changes of mood would be taken as signs of barbarism and immaturity.

It is also rather likely that many adult sexual attitudes of the sixteenth and early seventeenth centuries would be considered immature, irresponsible, and even infantile today. Elias only hints at these matters when discussing "behavior in the bedroom" and "relations between the sexes," but later authors have paid more attention to specifically sexual behavior in the narrow sense. The first important study, devoted to "the child and family life under the Ancien Régime," was written in French by Philippe Ariès in 1960 and translated in English as *Centuries of Childhood*.[4] Ariès, who apparently did not know Elias's earlier work, and who approached his subject simply as a historian, nevertheless comes to similar conclusions and, indeed, offers ample new illustrating material for their support. He, too, describes the gradual replacement of largely external controls by individual self-control, the transformation of social pressure exerted from without into moral pressure felt from within. This development at the same time created a growing gap between the worlds of adults and children. The historical forces that, over several centuries, eventually produced the inner-directed modern adult also led to the "discovery of childhood" as a special, separate, long period of preparation and inculcation.

Historically speaking, it took a long time before childhood, and later adolescence, could be perceived as delicate phases of a hazardous psychological development. This attitude first appeared in the upper social classes of the fifteenth and sixteenth centuries, but it was not before the mid-eighteenth century that it began to permeate all of society. Its eventual acceptance seems to have been furthered by two major factors: a change in the family structure and the growth of educational institutions outside the family.

Ariès provides a great deal of evidence that until well into the seventeenth century an intimate, protected family life was unknown. All family activities were part of a larger social life. The family was always open to the community and its influences. Even the wealthy did not live in sheltered private homes but rather in big houses, which were semipublic places, combining unspecified living quarters with guest rooms, servants lodgings, workshops, and offices. In these houses space for various work and leisure activities was created according to need, beds were set up and furniture was moved according to the fluctuating structure of the household. A constant flow of visitors, business partners, customers, officials, relatives, neighbors, and friends kept everyone in touch with the world at large.

Since life in these houses offered no privacy, the relationships between family members were not much closer than those with outsiders. Parents and children kept an emotional distance, addressing each other as "my son," "my daughter" and "Sir," "Madam"(or in French "Monsieur," "Madame," and in German "Herr Vater," "Frau Mutter"). Noble children in England called their parents "Mylord" and "Mylady." The use of the now familiar "Papa" and "Mamma," first names, or nicknames did not occur until the late seventeenth century.(After 1800 the English changed their spelling to "Mama," while the Americans used "Momma" and later simply spoke of "Mom" and "Dad.") To the extent that children could command parental attention, it consisted mainly of exhortation and punishment. After all, since infant mortality was high, parents were not very much inclined to grow closely attached to every newborn child. At any rate, even in the seventeenth century, children usually did not spend many years "in the bosom of the family." As infants, they were often given away to wet nurses and later brought up by domestics. Between the ages of seven and fourteen they normally left the house to become servants or apprentices in another household. Sons of noblemen became pages at the court of some other noble family.

This pattern changed only gradually with the emergence of a new type of family, which first became recognizable in the upper and middle classes of the late seventeenth century and went on to dominate the eighteenth century. It is a family type much closer to our contemporary notions than its predecessors, and it has recently provoked a considerable amount of research. For example, it had been described as the "closed domesticated nuclear family" by Lawrence Stone, who, in 1977, published a brilliant and comprehensive study concerning *The Family, Sex and Marriage in England 1500-1800*.[5] Stone once more confirmed the findings of Elias and Ariès and offered many new observations about specifically sexual behavior during the period in question. By consulting and interpreting church and court records, public and private documents, letters, and especially diaries, he was able to give us a realistic and startling impression of changing sexual attitudes among our distant forebears.

As far as the care of children is concerned, these attitudes clearly become more protective. As husbands and wives began to cherish their privacy and to cultivate their feelings for each other, boys and girls also turned into tender objects of affection. A new intimacy and emotional warmth began to develop in the increasingly isolated home, which slowly turned into a shelter, a haven secure from the world, an idyllic place free from all evil public influences. In the dawning Age of Enlightenment, children began to be seen as capable of reaching human perfection, provided they recieved the proper guidance and were shielded from the prevailing general social corruption. Of course, this idea at first put more responsibility on the parents, but eventually it also helped to diminish their role. Relatively soon the task of educating the young came to be regarded as so difficult and perilous that it required the full-time work of professionals. Accordingly, Stone also provides evidence for the second great source of change in adult-child relationships: the growth of educational enterprises and institutions, the origin of modern pedagogy.

However, public pedagogy remains a side issue in Stone's work. A more specific and detailed study of education in the eighteenth and nineteenth centuries was undertaken by the German author Rutschky under the title *Black Pedagogy, Sources Relating to the Natural History of Bourgeois Education* (1977).[6]

Rutschky's source collection illustrates how the new educational institutions developed out of monastic precedents and how first university colleges and later boarding schools put more and more emphasis on student discipline. By the same token, the teachers were increasingly held responsible not only for the correct transmission of knowledge but also for the correct moral training of their pupils. This moral training, in turn, eventually came to mean sexual repression.

In accordance with this trend, schools took on a quasi-military character. Like new recruits, the children were considered human raw material, which had to be formed into an effective army of productive citizens. Architecturally, educational institutions began to resemble barracks with large dormitories, washrooms, and latrines. The classrooms, often with windows close to the ceiling, allowed no view of the outside world or any other distraction. The students' benches were neatly lined up in rows facing the teacher, who sat on an elevated podium — an unquestioned higher authority.

Needless to say, such physical arrangements allowed for the total control of children as envisioned by antimasturbation crusaders such as Oest and Campe. Indeed, in the course of time, considerable refinements were introduced. Manufacturers of school benches, for example, offered new models that made any crossing of the legs impossible and, at the same time, gave teachers a clear view of the student's lower body. In the dormitories, the light was left burning so as the aid in the nocturnal supervision and prevention of self-abuse. Cold showers became standard practice in many institutions as did the routine inspection of bed sheets and clothing for "suspicious" stains. In short, from the physical layout and management of space and equipment to the psychological content of the curriculum, the sustained, organized prevention of masturbation became a major, not-so-secret agenda of most schools.

As Rutschky's collection demonstrates, pedagogical writings of the late eighteenth and the nineteenth centuries abound with advice on how to gain the upper hand on children by preventing their "self-abuse" or, at least, by turning it into a problem. The authors recommend not only that children be deliberately misinformed about their bodily functions and the process of reproduction but also that they be infibulated or fitted with chastity belts or similar contraptions. Of course, some of this advice was directed towards parents, but much of it was clearly aimed at professional educators and school administrators. Indeed, it is striking how often in these texts the parents appear as unfit for their task and as unwitting agents of their children's downfall. Over and over again, the new pedagogues criticizes the "excessive" love of mothers who touch, caress, and indulge their young at every opportunity and thereby weaken their moral fiber. Thus, it becomes obvious that the intimacy that arose within the closed, domesticated, nuclear family was seen as a threat by the professional institutions, who began to claim the ultimate control over education. Moreover, in contrast to the simple family home, they were able to marshal an abundant pedagogical arsenal against the spontaneity of the children in their care.

This does not mean that the schools increased or even insisted on corporal punishment. Indeed, very often the opposite was the case. The enlightened educators recognized fairly early that simple negative physical intervention was ineffective and counterproductive in the long run. Instead, every effort was made to gain control over the student's psyche. Frequent moral appeals, the cultivation of informants, intimate counseling sessions, philosophical walks, oral and written essays, confessions, and testimonials were used to discover all secrets of the young soul. The body, on the other hand, was no longer influenced so much by the whip and the rod as by a carefully calculated diet, cold baths, special clothing, furniture, and orthopedic devices. Finally, a special, new educational technology was developed to shape young sensibilities, perceptions, and movements. Beds, chairs, desks, blackboards, posters, games, toys, blocks, balls, sticks, and gymnastic equipment furthered a certain upright posture, measured responses, and a proper physical bearing. Tests, files, and report cards began to keep track of each student's progress in writing. Furthermore, the whole school year, each semester, month, week, day, and hour was planned and firmly scheduled in advance, with each lesson, exercise, walk, mealtime, and rest period detailed to the minute. In short, potentially (and in many cases actually) the school turned into a total institution.

The rise of such institutions in modern times has been exhaustively studied by Michel Foucault, who has written several books tracing the history of insane asylums[7] and prisons.[8] His findings with regard to these once unknown and now so familiar establishments also largely apply to schools. By analyzing a great variety of original sources (court records, legal codes, pamphlets, reports, medical and criminological textbooks, surveys, statistics, architectural studies, etc.), Foucault was able to show how, beginning in the seventeenth century, the will and ability to control not only the outward behavior but also the inner life of the population grew by leaps and bounds. The founding and rapid development of penal, psychiatric, and pedagogic institutions in the eighteenth and nineteenth centuries reflect the increasing thoroughness and sophistication with which the secular authorities shored up their position. "Proper education" became an essential element in the strategy of domesticating a potentially rebellious populace. People were seen as naturally good, but unruly, and therefore had to be taught early to develop a civilized self-control. This self-control, in turn, was essentially nothing more than the internalized social imperative as defined by the professionals. This is the reason why prisons, asylums, and schools not only expanded but also closed themselves off from society. At first, prisoners, patients, and students had freely received visitors or even had friends or relatives living with them for longer or shorter periods of time, but eventually all contact with the outside world was eliminated. The old universal social obligations of education, spiritual guidance, and punishment turned into pedagogy, psychiatry, and penology — new, highly specialized, and pure professional enterprises that were not to be contaminated or diluted by a meddling lay public. Thus, in the schools for example, the traditional, spontaneous, non guided means of socialization and intellectual stimulation were reduced to a single, well-defined curriculum. Parents, friends, neighbors, and other uncontrollable role models were relegated to the status of outsiders. For the professional educator the ideal child had no relatives, no past, and no social connections to anything beyond the school walls. It was a *tabula rasa*.

Numerous original sources show how much the new educators were disturbed by anything contradicting this image, such as unsolicited physical expressions or urges on the part of their students.

Youth and Sex in Modern Western Societies

Indeed, some pedagogical writings declared all fidgeting, mimicking, yawning, giggling, crying, bragging, daydreaming, and similar behavior to be symptomatic of "pedagogical pathology," i.e. psychological diseases of childhood. These were assumed to be more than three times as common as the physical childhood diseases, their number confirming, *ex negativo,* the great preponderance of the mind over the body. Accordingly, extensive lists of these pathologies were drawn up, ranging from nervousness and forgetfulness to rudeness and curiosity. Needless to say, there was only one cure: a longer and more intensive education.

This is the context in which the fight against childhood masturbation and the eventual denial of infantile sexuality during the last two centuries must be seen. It is a complex, multifaceted, and confusing, but internally consistent civilizing process in which even seemingly progressive and liberal policies serve the ultimate goal of more effective repression. For instance, when, in the eighteenth century, "enlightened" writers demanded a better education for girls, they usually did so with a simple and strong argument: prevent the fair sex from falling into a life of degradation and crime. Properly educated females would not turn into whores and unwed mothers and would not end up on the scaffold for having aborted or killed their children. The choice was only between the classroom on the one hand and the brothel or prison on the other. The endangered girl's innocence had to be preserved by professionals who protected her against her own destructive sexual impulses. No thought was given to changing social attitudes and institutions or to bettering the legal position of illegitimate children and mothers. In short, nobody was really interested in doing anything constructive about prostitution and infanticide. These evils were invoked only to justify a further extension of pedagogical control.

The double-faced or paradoxical character of sexual repression in the modern age had not always been noticed by all observers. Indeed, that certain steps toward social liberation can, at the same time, also bring greater sexual restrictions is hard to accept for some Anglo-Saxon researches who are unfamiliar with dialectical thinking. In their mind, the industrial revolution somehow brought on a massive wave of neo-Puritanism and prudery culminating in a

Victorian conspiracy of silence about sex, which is now finally in the process of being broken.

However, as Foucault and the other previously mentioned authors have shown, the matter is not as simple as suggested by these cliches. In fact, in his newest work, *The History of Sexuality*,[9] Foucault argues that, far from being silent on sexual problems, the nineteenth century was exceedingly eloquent and inquisitive, creating a greater awareness of sex than had ever before existed. It then proceeded to manipulate this awareness, thereby expanding and controlling human sexual options at the same time.

By the same token, Foucault does not see the sexual "permissiveness" of our own century as the final triumph of reason over bigotry, but rather as a largely illusionary gain. While it is true that sexual needs have increasingly been recognized, they have also been molded and preshaped by society long before they can be felt by any new individual.

Thus, in Western societies today, the sexuality of the young is still a more dangerous subject than it was in the early seventeenth century. Modern writers such as Sigmund Freud (*Three Essays on the Theory of Sexuality*, 1905) and Albert Moll (*The Sexual Life of the Child,* 1912) rediscovered infantile sexuality for our times, but they also found it to be highly problematic. Long overdue recognition created new anxieties. That these anxieties have not resolved themselves even now is proven by the periodic modern crusades against child molesters, incestuous parents, lesbian mothers, homosexual teachers, and child pornographers. Modern parents who dared to follow the educational practices of Henri IV and his court would still be arrested, convicted, and imprisoned in Europe as well as in America.

This traditional, physical, and more obvious aspect of modern sexual repression tends to be neglected or overlooked by many observers of the contemporary scene. Yet, when it comes to practical cases such as the treatment of juveniles in educational, correctional, or psychiatric institutions, direct represssive measures are by no means a thing of the past. Thus, in an indirect challenge to Foucault's belief in the increased subtlety of sexual control, the social historians Aron and Kempf have recently offered a new study of the antisexual syndrome in France. Their still untranslated book entitled *The Penis and the Demoralization of the West*

(1979) again gives us the history of the human body as formed and perceived by modern civilization.[10] Examining novels, cookbooks, encyclopedias, health guides, fashions, children's magazines, and especially court records, the authors find ample evidence for the systematic attempt at control through direct physical intervention. As they see it, the nineteenth century bourgeoisie gave themselves political and moral legitimacy by denying their own spontaneous bodily urges and by channeling them into ever-narrowing "acceptable" outlets. For them the body had become an efficient, profit-generating machine; therefore, the habit of wasting semen through masturbation appeared just as scandalous as the notion of throwing money out of the window. The ferocity with which they persecuted "abnormal" sexual manifestations is understandable only against this background, and so is their concern with the early "normalization" of the young. Children and adolescents were, and still are, the test case for the success of all control strategies. In controlling its offspring, the bourgeoisie tried to control itself, or rather its future. Thus, the meaning of the taboo becomes clear: ultimately, the threat and temptation of infantile and adolescent sexuality helped to keep adult desires in check and to prevent a genuine sexual revolution.

Obviously, such a revolution still has not occurred, and the question of whether it is posssible or even desirable must await further study of our present situation before it can find an answer.

REFERENCES AND RECOMMENDED READING

1. Stone, Lawrence, *The Family, Sex and Marriage in England 1500-1800*, New York: Harper & Row, 1977, pp. 507-509.
2. Rutschky, Katharina, *Schwarze Pädagogik, Quellen zur Naturgeschichte der bürgerlichen Erziehung*. Frankfurt/M: Ullstein, 1977, pp. 304-315.
3. Elias, Norbert, *The Civilizing Process, The Development of Manners, Changes in the code of conduct and feeling in early modern times*. New York: Urizen Books, 1978.
4. Ariès, Philippe, *Centuries of Childhood*. New York: Knopf, 1962.
5. Stone, *op. cit.*
6. Rutschky, *op. cit.*
7. Foucault, Michel, *Madness and Civilization, A History of Insanity in the Age of Reason*. New York: Pantheon, 1965.
8. ———, *Discipline and Punish, The Birth of the Prison*. New York: Pantheon, 1977.

9. _____, *The History of Sexuality*, vol. I, *An Introduction*. New York: Pantheon, 1978.
10. Aron, Jean-Paul and Roger Kempf, *Le Pénis et la Démoralisation de l'Occident*. Paris: Bernard Grasset, 1979.

Chapter Two

CONTEMPORARY PATTERNS:
Emerging Issues of the Sexual Rights of Adolescents in Institutions

DIANE BLAKE BRASHEAR

ADOLESCENTS are institutionalized for many different reasons, and there is an institution to match virtually every reason. In spite of substantial differences among these various institutions, all of them face similar concerns about how to deal with the sexuality and sexual expression of the adolescents in their care. Who is responsible for dealing with these issues? What rights do institutionalized adolescents have? What should be done?

Outside of institutions there has been some obvious progress in educating parents and other authority figures so that some groups of teenagers are better served now than previously. The current alarming incidence of teen pregnancy and sexually transmitted disease has prompted adults to give teens more education and health services, at least in the areas of contraception and sexually transmitted diseases. While those parents and other adults who do not wish to address these problems are sometimes vocal, they usually avoid dealing with the issue by grudgingly allowing specialists to provide sex education and sexual health services.

A problem for adults dealing with institutionalized adolescents is that the adults are often in their jobs because of some vocational goal other than that of sex education — many of them are interested primarily in teaching the handicapped or rehabilitating youthful offenders, for example. Usually their professional training has not included sex education; yet, by the very nature of their contact with teens, they are the adults most likely to be on the front line in dealing with adolescent sexual concerns and behavior. Out of their own anxiety about sexual issues (often stemming from their lack of preparation), ambivalent and inconsistent responses to sexual behaviors naturally occur. One staff member may be permissive and supportive when confronted with adolescent anxiety about masturbation, while another may be punitive.

Staff members, in dealing directly with adolescent sexuality, may also be confronted with their own ambivalence about teenage sexual behaviors. For example, while they may understand intellectually that adolescence is a period of experimentation and sexual development, being directly confronted with two teens mutually masturbating may evoke emotional responses of shock and embarrassment — despite cognitive understandings. The very nature of institutionalization creates a situation where staff members may be privy to sexual behaviors that the non institutionalized adolescent may also be doing, but more privately and secretly. Because the staff is vested with some authority, they may feel more compelled to do something about the sexual behavior.

Another complicating factor is that the staff's role is often one of corrector or trainer. How does that role affect the staff member's repertoire of responses to the adolescent's sexual behavior? Any adult or peer is, whether he or she wants to be or not, a sex educator. What is the appropriate response? Should it be an individual one or an official policy? What if the institution's official response to a sexual behavior conflicts with an individual staff member's personal attitude?

To have sexual issues develop between staff and institutionalized adolescents is complex and confusing in itself. The situation is further complicated by the lack of clear definition of what the official institutional response should be. First of all, the institutions and the reasons why teens are there vary greatly. In voluntary institutions, e.g. a school for the deaf, parents often give their child to an educational boarding institution yet theoretically hold authority for those moral guidelines they wish to impart to their child. Should the school administration feel obligated to follow known parental guidelines, even in the face of risk to the health of the individual? For instance, should the institution withhold contraceptives from a sexually active female whose parents refuse to acknowledge such behavior? Or does the school administration view the teenager as legally responsible for his or her own behavior and act accordingly, thereby threatening the school-parent relationship, which is valuable if the teen is to stay active in the total institutional program.

Another consideration is how sex education is defined by various institutions. There are often major differences. For example, in an institution for deaf adolescents a sex education process might involve an information-awareness-discussion process where the student becomes the integrator of his or her own knowledge. This method is vastly different from that of a school for retarded persons that offers instruction with defined, acceptable behaviors and specific training, such as how to masturbate.

Consider, too, the correctional facility where youth are placed because of antisocial behavior. If they are voluntarily placed by parents, who has primary sex education authority? If the antisocial behavior itself is sexual (prostitution, for example), who is responsible — and for what? Often inmates in these institutions are more sexually experienced than the staff. Does experience substitute for sex education? What is the sex education process in an institution? Is it different than in the community outside? Do peer groups have more power and influence within institutions?

To be more specific, the following seem to be key relevant questions:

1. What is the institution's official policy on sexual learning and behaviors? Does this vary based on the nature of the institution, its goals and legal responsibilities? How is this policy determined?
2. What role should the staff play as they have informal access to students' sexual learning? How does this role fit with administration policy?
3. What rights do adolescents in institutions have to obtain sexual learning and health care and to establish their own behaviors? Do they forfeit these rights in some cases? What role does the institution have in insuring these rights?

Until recently, it has appeared that many institutions, staffs, and communities have begged the questions. By not doing anything there has been a groundswell of sexual problems, concerns, and incidents that are often handled on a piecemeal basis. This approach, while resolving nothing, has helped to keep things from getting completely out of hand, has bought everybody time, and has saved them the discomfort of initiating the social changes necessary to address the real problems of institutionalized adolescents. Now it is time to be realistic. We cannot continue to avoid and resist. Recognition of these issues by professionals, advocates for adolescent sexual rights, and the adolescents themselves is forcing the question. The adolescents are the most demanding force. As their sexual concerns and behaviors become more apparent, the only responsibile approach for the institution is to respond. The following four areas are obviously in need of specific response.

Sex Education

SIECUS (The Sex Information and Education Council of the United States), founded in 1964 by professionals who recognized the need for sexual learning advocates, has long maintained that all human beings are sexual persons who need to know about their sexuality. While grandly stated concepts are important as support, the following case illustrates the general point more graphically. An obese thirteen year old girl delivered a 7lb. 6oz. baby boy in her dormitory bed. She thought her stomach was upset, and the houseparent suggested that she rest. The young mother didn't know how this happened, i.e. she didn't know about sexual intercourse. The houseparent didn't know how it happened either. Oh, the houseparent knew about sexual intercourse, but she didn't think the thirteen year old was mature or attractive enough to be sexually active. This event happened in 1979. Ask any person who works with teens and he or she will tell you that the dissonance between what adolescents are experiencing and what they know is so ridiculous that we adults frequently reject it as being too absurd to be true. Teenagers face much anxiety that comes from the dilemma of being sexually provoked through peer and community pressures on the one hand and the widespread lack of information on the other. One fifteen year old said "I didn't think when I was young that I had any choice. If a guy wanted you, you let him."

We know that adolescents are sexually stimulated and active; even the most conservative reports recognize this. Those who work with institutionalized teens know that just being in a more controlled environment does not stop the problem — or deal with it either.

It does not make any sense to defend sex education based on pregnancy and venereal disease scares. The most important reason for sex education is that the adolescent needs to have the chance to develop biologically, psychologically, and experientially so that sexual opportunity and behavior are present. Sexual learning opportunities are as important to a young person's full development as learning to read and write. Often, staff members seem so frightened by this responsibility for sexual learning that they fail to recognize the opportunities that institutionalization offers for meeting this responsibility. The staff, for example, has easy access to the adolescent, often in informal sexual learning opportunities such as the late night talk sessions between the houseparent and the resident.

As much as adolescents have a right to know, they also have a right to be sexual. Only through deliberate sexuality learning opportunities can we help them help themselves in their sexual development. The fifteen year old young woman mentioned earlier learned to say no when she discovered, via small group discussion, that there were other options. Education that focuses just on genitals only reforces genital behavior as *the* only sexual option. Education that focuses on sexuality helps individuals recognize and experience a broader range of sexual expression.

It would be a cop-out merely to say that institutionalized adolescents should have sex education. Most professionals recognize this. The emerging issue in sex education is not whether to do it but who does it and how. Do special populations require special treatment and approaches? What are the administrative and political ramifications? What strategies should be planned to insure the integration of sexual learning into institutional programs? How does one deal with resistance?

We must advocate social change planning as an integral part of providing sex education. Without planning that takes into account the practical issues of social change that will occur (that a birth control clinic will be necessary, for example), no sex education will last. Sex education, because it touches so many individuals so profoundly, really is social change, change in attitudes and behaviors, and the ramifications throughout the social system will be powerful. They will be especially powerful within a more closed system, such as an institution for adolescents. Social systems knowledge and change theory are as important in sex education programs as the program content.

One effective program that paid careful attention to systems knowledge and change theory occurred in a state-administered school for the physically handicapped. Professional staff, alarmed by pregnancies and more open sexual behaviors, agreed they wanted sex education for the school. That was all they agreed upon; they didn't know who, what, or how. Before they attempted to answer these questions, they developed a broader plan that included a staff course in human sexuality; a questionnaire that was distributed after the course to find out whether all staff (teachers, houseparents, administrators) wanted sex education for the students; an advisory committee of parents, sex education experts, and community and religious leaders; and development of curriculum and a pilot project. It took two years, but that school had its own effective program, a program with broad-based support that allowed the necessary social change to occur. Contrast this with the once or twice a year visits from the local Planned Parenthood educator who, while competent, carries the full burden of being the sex educator.

Sexual Medical Health Care

Recently, the director of a large treatment center for adolescent girls was asked how abortion was handled. "It isn't," she answered. "I'm too afraid to deal with it since we get state money. So I let Planned Parenthood do sex education and the health center handles the pregnant girls." The reality is that many of these girls are pregnant and have no option other than carrying the baby full term. If they weren't institutionalized, abortion might be an option.

Traditionally, in the eyes of the law, minors (adolescents) have been subjected to many inequities, the most dramatic of which is their right to effective control of their own bodies. Under common law, children were treated as the property of their parents. Many of those same laws are in effect today, regulating such matters as a minor's right to enter into a contract, marry, and execute a will. In the area of medical treatment, which is of vital importance in regard to sexual rights, minors often cannot receive medical treatment without parental consent. In many situations, a physician giving medical treatment without consent of the parents is subject to legal actions by the parents. There are, of course, exceptions to that practice. These include such circumstances as an emancipated minor or an emergency endangering the life or health of the minor. Many states have lowered the age of consent to medical treatment to eighteen and have also allowed even younger adolescents to receive medical care for sexually transmitted disease and/or pregnancy. The Supreme Court decisions on abortion now lend support to providing contraceptives to minors without parental consent.

If an institutionalized adolescent requires medical treatment, a number of problems surface. If parental consent is necessary in the state, who gives that consent, the parent or the institution? If there are no legal restrictions, do institutionalized adolescents have the right to exercise their freedom to consent to medical treatment?

Generally, the parents of an adolescent in a more voluntary type of institution, e.g. a school for the deaf or blind or voluntary commitment to a hospital, sign a form allowing the institution's authorities to give consent for medical treatment. In those cases where the youth are sent to an institution by a court order, the institution becomes responsible for the care and treatment of those teenagers. In a sense, the court orders the institution to become substitute parents. In those states where consent is required for medical treatment, the institutionalized adolescent is unable to receive treatment without the knowledge and consent of someone in that institution.

Institutionalized adolescents who do not need adult permission for medical treatment are at first sight certainly in a better position. However, usually there are institutional rules restricting free movement off the grounds of the institution. These restrictions are necessary in many cases. The situation results, though, in the adolescent having a right (to consent to his or her own medical treatment) but not being able to exercise it. Essentially, this results in denying that right.

Adolescents in institutions that have legal control over them (correctional schools, for example) are not allowed to consent to medical treatment, although the institution itself is permitted to give such consent. Yet, these institutionalized individuals are also often denied the right of sexual medical health care because the institution refuses to provide such care for fear of community or parental reprisals. In short, adequate sexual health care is not available because the staff refuses to permit it.

Regulation of Private Sexual Behavior

Perhaps no one sexual issue is frought with so many unanswered questions as the issue of privacy. Observation and control of sexual behaviors that are normative to individuals create inhibition and embarrassment for the adolescent. At a developmental period when self-image is so vulnerable and body concepts so critical, privacy is of great importance to the teenager. Yet, where can the institutionalized youth go to be alone? If one has trouble finding a place to be alone to read and daydream, where will he or she be able to privately explore his or her own body, to fantasize?

The opportunity for experimentation in same-sex and other sex behaviors is even more of an issue. Because privacy is so difficult to provide in an institutional setting, should a greater amount of such experimentation be permitted in public than would be tolerated if a teenager had easy access to such traditionally private places as the back seat of a car? Who decides how much is too much? If younger children are also in the institution, what effect does the adolescents' behavior have on them? Is it positive? Should the institution make greater efforts to provide more privacy for the residents?

Finding socially appropriate forms of sexual expression is a complex task that requires a sense of discrimination and cognitive skill on the part of the searcher. Often the institutionalized adolescent lacks that discriminatory skill — that may be why he or she is in the institution — yet he or she still has a need for privacy and sexual expression. A staff, comfortable and innovative in providing sexual learning, can help teenagers to develop ways to privately express their sexuality as well as ways that are socially appropriate in public situations. Institutional staff often have frequent opportunities to use real-life situations for social-sexual learning rather than having to rely on more indirect situations, such as those presented during discussions, lectures, and films. Often a simple permission-giving statement — "Touching yourself feels good but keep the door closed so you can do it privately" — can be quite effective.

A dilemma in the privacy issue is the institutional regulations that are enforced presumably to guard against antisocial behavior. Always keeping doors open, always needing to be with a buddy while on campus, receiving physical exams and medical care in a large open room — practices of this sort may be practical in institutional management, but they can also be so dehumanizing as to be more damaging to the adolescent than helpful or protective.

Homosexualities

It is fairly well accepted among professionals (at least on a cognitive level) that adolescents will engage in same-sex fantasies and behaviors. How such behavior is treated is very important to the sexual development of the adolescent. Homophobia, especially in males, can inhibit sexual development and create serious psychological conflict.

This is a sensitive area for several reasons. For one, there are homosexual adolescents. What happens when their behavior is denied or labeled as experimental when, in truth, they need to explore their feelings about their sexual identity and self-image? On the other hand, if the individual really is experimenting, how will this exploration affect him or her? What were the circumstances under which the sexual experience developed? Important, how is the peer group responding to same-sex feelings and behaviors if they become known? During adolescence, fear of homosexuality, fear of being so different, can be a ruling force and inhibit expressions of intimacy among same sex friends. These relationships are already intensified by virtue of the individuals being together in an institution. In such living situations, which serve same-sex adolescents, intimacy is often sought and expressed through same-sex relationships that have sexual components but usually are a replacement for the love and caring that are missing in most institutional care.

The need for closeness and intimacy, for touching and warmth, is a basic human need. At the extreme, infants who do not have these needs met die. One way to have these intimacy needs met is through sexual behavior.

During puberty, there are normal impulses to experiment sexually. These impulses, coupled with intimacy needs, can be very powerful and overwhelming. Teenagers living at home may have a fairly good opportunity to have their intimacy needs met through contact with their families and private expression with friends. Yet, the intimacy needs of the institutionailized adolescent are almost universally ignored. These persons are separated from their families, often for traumatic or extremely problematic reasons. Initially then, they usually are not getting the quality contact with other people necessary to satisfy their intimacy needs. In addition, if the entire area of their sexual needs is ignored, they are quite vulnerable to same sex activities that may or may not have occurred were they not institutionalized.

In identifying emerging sexual issues related to adolescents in institutions, the intent is not to create more anxiety and confusion — the treatment of sexual issues is anxiety producing enough. It is, however, important to recognize that these sexual issues are very complex with no single right or wrong resolution. There are few prescriptions that will satisfactorily answer any of these concerns. If there is an area where pioneer efforts are needed and welcome, this is it. It is going to be a tough job, requiring skill, compassion, commitment, and risk. The opportunities are exciting, and the challenge is important enough to risk faltering and even some failure. We can hardly do less since the institutionalized adolescents themselves are facing an even greater risk: irreparable harm to their social development.

Often when we think of institutions, we tend to group all the humans in them into neat categories: the retarded, the handicapped, the delinquent, and so on. In doing so, we have taken a step toward dehumanizing these young people. Dealing with their sexual rights and responsibilities is a step in the opposite direction — and one way of keeping us all human.

Chapter Three

THE INSTITUTIONALIZED ADOLESCENT AND THE ETHICS OF DESEXUALIZATION

GERALD J. MURPHY

THE purpose of this chapter is to identify some critical issues regarding institutionalization and to discuss their impact upon the psychosexual development of adolescents in long-term, residential programs. Specifically, we are interested in examining moral and ethical implications in the way institutions deal with sex and sexuality and how these residential programs shape and determine the way young people come to feel, think, and behave as sexual human beings.

Some terms and concepts, however, need to be defined and discussed at the outset. The key words in this chapter are *institutionalization, adolescent, sex, sexuality, desexualization* and *ethics*. These terms require some definition since they are not self-explanatory, and their use can often convey different meanings to the reader.

- *Institutionalization* is a process that fosters excessive dependency upon group norms and behaviors and generally results in poorly developed self-identity, inadequate reality testing, and other-directed behavior.
- *Adolescence* is defined by *Webster's New Collegiate Dictionary* as "the state or process of growing up."[1] Understood as a transition from childhood to adulthood, adolescence is a social invention; it is not a biological process as, for instance, puberty is. Puberty just happens; adolescence must be acquired.[2]

- *Sex* is a word that is synonymous with intercourse in our culture. It is the act of sexual union of a male and a female, in which the penis is inserted into the vagina.*
- *Sexuality* implies more than intercourse and the pursuit of erotic pleasure. It involves the need for love and personal fulfillment. The sexuality of men and women is regarded today as an important aspect of personality and essential in enhancing communication and intimacy.[3]
- *Desexualization* is a process whereby development of personality, communication, and intimacy in heterosocial situations is either denied or excessively controlled by administrative, staff, and organizational forces.
- *Ethics* refers to the moral quality of a course of action. It assumes that there are rules or standards that govern the way residential programs for adolescents are to be administered and that such standards must not lead to any physical, emotional, psychological, sexual, and social harm of residents. Ethics is action oriented. It looks at behavior and judges whether the conduct is right or good in light of moral principles accepted in the wider community.

The institutional life of many adolescents in long-term residential programs raises a number of ethical issues regarding their rights to develop as sexual human beings. That nearly half a million adolescents in long-term institutions may differ significantly from one another in terms of physical, emotional, mental, and social conditions and that the care institutions themselves, therefore, serve very different needs is no reason to deny that some common forces operate in nearly all institutions of care for children and adolescents in the United States and that these forces often have a potentially harmful effect on the sexual health and well-being of their residents.

The Structural Environment and Desexualization

The process of institutionalization usually begins by segregating the sexes and communalizing individuals within same-sex settings. In these situations group norms and rules prevail, and individuals are expected to behave in ways that are fairly uniform

---

* For an extended discussion of the terms *sex, sexuality, and sexual behavior*, see Erwin J. Haeberle's *The Sex Atlas*. New York: The Seabury Press, 1978, pp. 125-127.

and predictable. The structural environment of a typical institution for adolescents is deliberately designed so as to assure adequate supervisory control over the day-to-day behavior of its residents. Administrative, staff, and organizational needs and constraints pose a constant threat to any effort that attempts to administer programs "in the best interest of the child."

An institutionalized adolescent is a product of any long-term institution that has socialized a youngster according to its own administrative needs. These adolescents operate in a passive and dependent manner rather than in an assertive and independent one. Personal identity is largely swallowed up by group indentity, and the young person understandably exhibits traits indicative of low self-esteem and poor reality testing. Clinically, the institutionalized adolescent presents a picture of depressive personality.

Institutions for adolescents may vary greatly in terms of the needs they address and the services they render, but they are all, for the most part, desexualized and desexualizing environments. In the first place they are desexualized because they segregate the sexes and create exclusively homosocial environments of peers. This same-sex grouping of adolescents takes place without the consent of the young male and female and generally stays imposed upon the individual throughout all the years that the person is institutionalized. An institution may, therefore, be characterized as a desexualized environment to the extent that it segregates the sexes involuntarily and prevents a meaningful communication to take place between them.

Second, institutions are desexualizing environments in the sense that predominately sex-negative attitudes and behaviors on the part of administrations and staff often prevent the growth and development of a healthy sexual self-awareness among their residents. Sex education is rarely found among institutional programs for adolescents, and sex counseling is provided mostly for these youngsters who become sexually active and are therefore in need of contraceptive information. The message that sex and sexuality are somehow "dirty" prevails; consequently, little if any effort is made to develop in adolescent residents of long-term care facilities attitudes, knowledge, and skills regarding sexuality that will enhance the sense of themselves as sexual human beings who are capable of communicating their needs to others to establish and sustain warm, close, and intimate relationships. The sex-negative modelling on the part of staff in terms of their disapproving attitudes and behaviors engenders anxiety and fears regarding sexual relationships while fostering greater dependency upon group life and activities. The institutionalized adolescent is, by definition, also a desexualized adolescent.

The Interpersonal Environment and Desexualization

There are many structural elements of institutionalization that adversely affect the psychosexual development of adolescent residents. Among these are same-sex groupings; priority of group norms and activities and emphasis on uniform and predictable behavior; absence of sex education programs; and a generally sex-negative attitude on the part of administrators and staff. In addition, adolescent residents of long-term institutions have to contend with an interpersonal environment that is desexualizing. Such an environment denies residents a basic right to privacy, distorts the reality of heterosocial relationships, manipulates and stigmatizes sexual expression, and provides inadequate sexual role models for the youngsters in its care.

Although privacy is a basic human right and is recognized as an essential condition for developing and maintaining close, caring, and intimate relationships, it is the one thing that institutions tend to ignore. Since an institution is understood as a public place (whether it is a hospital, orphanage, or dentention home) that requires round-the-clock supervision, the idea of residents having a private place and private time is difficult for staff to accept and respect. This seems true even for those institutions which, as a matter of policy and staff commitment, attempt to provide a certain degree of privacy for their residents. Even if the rights to privacy receive the strongest administrative and staff support, the residents may continue to fear intrusion simply because they do not have control over the situation and circumstances.

The problem of assuring some privacy to residents of long-term care institutions is dramatized by the following incident, which recently occurred in a large, metropolitan, progressive, rehabilitation hospital. A young quadriplegic male had been married to another quadriplegic patient for six months, and both were living in private quarters at the hospital. The staff believed that everything was going well for the couple until one day the husband let the counselor know that he and his wife had not engaged in any sexual activity the whole six months of their marriage. The couple was simply afraid that if they attempted to have sex it would take them a good deal of time, and they feared that some staff person would inadvertently enter their rooms and embarrass them! Fear, guilt, and embarrassment kept this couple from informing staff of their problems. They felt hopeless and helpless.

The homosocial environment of most institutions tends also to distort the sexual attitudes of residents toward members of the other sex, and this frequently leads to inappropriate heterosexual behavior. A same-sex grouping easily lends itself to sexist attitudes wherein males tend to view females as primarily sex objects who exist for the male's pleasure. Young adolescent females in sex-segregated institutions, on the other hand, tend to idealize and romanticize sexual relationships, viewing the male as a source of safety and protection. The segregation of the sexes, combined with an official conspiracy of silence regarding sexuality, inevitably breeds ignorance and misinformation regarding this aspect of life and tends to create confusion, uncertainty, misunderstanding, and conflict in establishing relationships with members of the other sex.

A more subtle, but nevertheless harmful, effect of the interpersonal environment of institutions upon adolescent residents has to do with the manipulation of sexuality and the stigmatization of sexual expression. Manipulation occurs in the attempt of staff to frustrate residents from developing close relationships with peers of the same sex or other sex by requiring communal and closely supervised activities.

Gestures of mutual affection and caring among residents are strongly discouraged, and such behaviors as touching, holding hands, hugging, kissing, and/or being alone with a friend are generally held in check by the effective use of group pressure and a prevailing sexist attitude toward appropriate male/female behavior. The stigmatization of sexual expression follows from such a repressive climate in that masturbatory activity is generally not acknowledged as a normal, healthy behavior, and intercourse is considered as something dirty for teenagers to do. Homosexually oriented adolescents suffer the greatest pain, since the sex-negative attitude in most institutions continues to view such behavior as being sick and depraved.

In considering the impact of the interpersonal environment upon the sexuality of adolescent residents, it is important also to examine the relationship between staff and youngsters in terms of role models. In many instances, institutions fail to train staff to respond to residents in ways that address their specific needs and that model appropriate sex behaviors. It is not uncommon, in residential programs for adolescent boys, for female staff to act in ways that succeed in controlling residents' behavior without recognizing that such behavior can create hostile attitudes toward women. Some roles that female staff tend to play are those of mother, seducer, and/or castrator. On the other hand, male staff in institutions for boys may assume the role of sargeant, peer, and/or seducer. All such roles for staff are highly inappropriate because they manipulate the younger person, distort relationships between adults and teens, and may even adversely affect development of gender identity and sexual orientation.

What Can Institutions Do?

This discussion has focused on elements of institutionalization that negatively affect the way adolescent residents think, feel, and behave as sexual human beings. It is not so much that life in an institution per se causes psychosexual problems; it is, rather, a matter of how a given institution is administratively and programmatically organized and to what extent sex-negative attitudes and behaviors prevail.

If institutions "institutionalize" their adolescent residents, then desexualization inevitably occurs. Healthy psychosexual development requires an environment that supports an individual's rights to express legitimate needs and to attempt to fulfill these needs in ways consistent with one's own well-being and that of others. Institutionalized adolescents are young people whose own psychosocial and psychosexual needs have been subordinated to administrative and organizational policies, rules, and practices. They are children who have been stripped of freedom, denied privacy, deprived of intimacy, and given not a name but a case number for a personality.

Administrators and staff in many institutions for adolescents throughout the United States might quite predictably consider this analysis of how institutions deal with human sexuality as harsh and, perhaps, even unfair. In the first place, institutions exist to serve special populations with special needs. To meet these needs, round-the-clock supervision and communal programs are essential. Second, such an environment does not inevitably lead to desexualization — many institutional staff may exclaim, "our program certainly does not!" On this basis of this reasoning, staff and administrators may be tempted to accept desexualization as occurring somewhere else, but not in their own institution.

Lest all of us who work in institutions for adolescents be guilty of seeing the speck in a fellow institution's eye while failing to see the beam in our own, certain rights of adolescents living in institutions can be identified, which can then serve as a measuring yard to assess how well any institution, regardless of its purpose and function, is preventing the insidious process of institutionalization from taking hold of its residents. In the context of these basic rights, the responsibility of institutions to protect, develop, enhance, and sustain the psychosexual development of its adolescent residents can briefly be discussed.

Some basic rights of adolescents in institutions are as follows:

1. The right to respect from administrators and staff.
2. The right to privacy.
3. The right to an education.
4. The right to worship.
5. The right to receive counseling and guidance.
6. The right to receive adequate services to meet special needs.
7. The right to participate in decisions affecting one's life.
8. The right to visit with close relatives and friends.
9. The right to a safe and secure environment.
10. The right to be discharged from a program as soon as conditions and circumstances permit.

As is the case with all principles that guide conduct, these abstract rights need to be applied to special populations of youngsters in very different and, perhaps, highly specialized institutions. The moral and ethical implications of sexuality as they relate to the retarded in institutions[4] might differ considerably in terms of specific conditions and circumstances than they would, perhaps, with adolescent residents of a group home. Nevertheless, the rights of patients and/or residents in all institutions — even juvenile detention homes — remain essentially the same, and the ethical implications of how well institutional programs and practices address these needs can and must be continually assessed by all concerned parties: the professional administrators and mental health workers, child care workers, and the families of adolescents in institutions.

The rights of adolescents in institutions suggest ways in which administrators and staff could begin to examine their institution's approach to psychosexual development and its expression among their young residents. Keeping in mind that sexuality relates to personality and that a person's growth in sexual self-awareness is closely connected with one's ability to communicate and share intimacy with others, an institution should be able to find appropriate ways to —

1. show residents respect;
2. guarantee some acceptable degree of privacy;
3. provide sufficient sex education;
4. offer guidance and counseling;
5. permit a reasonable amount of heterosocial contacts;
6. welcome residents' input into decision making regarding many of these same issues;
7. address the special sexual concerns of their residents within the constraints of the institution's purpose, function, and available resources.

It is, after all, not a question in many instances of adding on additional programs and services so much as doing a better job in carrying out already existing ones. Changes in attitudes and role behavior of staff as well as changes in unduly restrictive policies and practices are not additional burdens. Indeed, once effected and carried out so that the "best interest of the child" is more genuinely being served, the acknowledged burden and responsibility of administrators and staff may shift to a point where, if not appreciably decreased, it will appear less weighty. When doing their best for youth committed to their care, administrators and staff of institutions can make their own the motto that motivates and sustains the efforts of Father Flanagan's Boys Town: "He's not heavy; he's my brother."

REFERENCES

1. *Webster's New Collegiate Dictionary.* Springfield, Mass.: G. and C. Merriam Co., 1979.
2. Somner, Barber Baker. *Puberty and Adolescence.* Oxford: Oxford University Press, 1978.
3. *Educational and Treatment in Human Sexuality: The Training of Health Professionals. Report of a WHO Meeting, Technical Reports Series 572.* Geneva: World Health Organization, 1975.
4. Narot, Rabbi Joseph R. "The Moral and Ethical Implications of Sexuality as They Relate to the Retarded" in *Human Sexuality and the Mentally Retarded,* edited by Felix de la Cruz and Gerald D. LaVeck. New York: Penguin Books, 1973.

PART II
MANAGEMENT OF SEXUAL BEHAVIOR

Chapter Four

ADMINISTRATIVE CONCERNS

Ord Matek

IN every residential institution, each individual who is a significant part of that program may differ on many counts from some or even all of the other persons who are part of that program. Each person brings his or her own life-style and life values into each decision. This conflict of values can flare up into serious staff disagreements in the form of personality clashes, or it may be continually discussed, clarified, and worked out where the need for doing so is recognized. The conflict, however, is inevitable.

Howard, thirteen years old and a resident of a small treatment institution, had only one momento of his father. It was an inexpensive watch that did not even keep good time, and Howard rarely wore it. In fact his feelings about it were ambivalent, because the relationship with his father was so emotionally charged. His father had been verbally and physically abusive of Howard and his sister for many years. In addition, the father had terrorized the sister into incestuous behavior. The father deserted the family and disappeared when the incest was reported to the police. Howard, who had learned about the sexual activity, was given the watch by his father as a bribe to be silent about the incest. Howard never did tell on the father; he was too frightened of him to do so. The watch, however, was the only gift he ever got from his father. It became a problem when Howard accidentally dropped it while getting some other items out of his desk drawer, where he kept the watch. It broke, and Howard was confused as to what to do next. He consulted each of the staff and some of his friends in the institution and got almost as many answers as there were people whom he asked. ("It's a cheap watch and it's not worth repairing."… "You don't have to decide right now. Let it set in the drawer till you are sure." . . . "It's the only tangible reminder of your father. Why not repair it for the sentimental meaning?". . . "You hate your father, why keep that reminder.". . .)

An institution can focus on some of the issues that represent conflicts of values, but there is no way that everyone can be prepared for and agreed on each aspect of group living and the progress for each resident at all times. Even where the answers come from the front office via administrative dicta, they cannot address everything; even then there remains the problem of individual interpretations of any order.

While this conflict of values is general, it is particularly pronounced in the realm of sexuality. Most people, including professionals, are generally not at ease in discussing sexual issues; there are frequently private reservations and disagreements that may not be aired but that are subtly or even openly acted on by individual staff as a reaction to their own sexual value system.

> Mary, an eighteen year old retarded girl, was evaluated by the psychologist employed by the insitution as not being truly sexually provocative even though a lot of her talk and behavior in the sheltered workshop was sexually explicit. Her history was that of worried parents who severely repressed her femininity out of their concern that she might be led into pregnancy. They dressed her in grotesque fashion and generally made her unattractive. The psychologist felt it made her feel unloved and unlovable. Her response, particularly in the workshop where she felt especially stifled, was to aggressively push for attention by engaging in explicit sexual language and flirtatious behavior. Staff were instructed not to react to these patterns and instead to tell Mary how well she was working (when she did so) and how attractive she now looked in her institution-bought clothes. Some staff could do so, but a large number were still affronted by her sexual language and behavior despite the staff meetings. They continued to react out of their personal orientation, unable to accept and implement the recommendations.[1]

With great effort and over time, a sensitive administration could address this kind of problem. It might not be in time for a unified approach to Mary, but it could be worked out in time for other Mary's who inevitably will follow. However, the longevity of staff employment is an obstacle. Staff turnover is often too rapid to allow for optimal staff training.

Redl talks about selecting staff who have "the ability to sacrifice what personal style . . . they happen to be most enamored with to the clinical strategy needed at a certain time".[2] He also differentitates among various types of institutions and recognizes that the above formulation is critical in a treatment institution but may not operate the same way in institutions with goals other than treatment. "One of the sharpest dividing lines between institutions with a primarily educational goal and treatment homes can be drawn around the concept of symptom tolerance".[2] Adolescents however, live in all types of institutions, and their very sexuality prompts a wide range of reactions from staff.

Even where symptom tolerance is stressed, it may present especially difficult problems to the administration of an institution when the symptoms reflect sexual phenomena. The community wherein the institution resides may not have any symptom tolerance for behaviors that the institution has learned to accept. The problem of an adolescent living in an institution who may engage in Peeping Tom activities in the community is an example. The institutional personnel may correctly see him as essentially harmless and may even feel he has made some first steps in the beginning control of his voyeurism. The community at large, however, may not be able to accept his presence in an open institution when they feel vulnerable because of him. Community standards may also be the guidelines that prompt parents to remove a youngster from a residential facility where he might have been voluntarily placed were they to discover that one of the staff was a homosexual, even though there may never have been a history of sexual interaction with young people on the part of the staff member. In fact, the particular staff member may have been particularly skilled and helpful to the program.

The long-time program director of one community living facility for retarded adolescents and young adults was summarily fired with no explanation when he was earlier observed by some of the institution's board members to have just emerged from a gay bar. He had previously recieved a new annual contract based on an evaluation, rating him at the highest level. None the less, despite the disruption to the program continuity, his dismissal was seen as justified by the majority of the parents of the residents as well as the board. (He subsequently filed a lawsuit for breach of contract.)

Parents of institutional residents have their own sexual norms, even though they may be very much at variance from one another. However, these norms may not readily fit into the institutional life-style. What, then, does the institution do? Shall it substitute its own ideas for those of the parent, or can it so individualize its residents that each has his or her life values affirmed? Actually neither is quite the case, but sometimes the dilemma is particularly dramatic.

>Janice, fifteen years old and in long-term hospital care due to chronic illness, came from a family that practiced nudism. They were ardent believers in the advantages of a totally unrestrained body open to the benefit of the elements. They went for frequent weekends and for vacations to nudist camps, and at home all of them often wore no clothes. Janice was comfortable with that life-style, but the adolescent group she became part of in the institution was not. Whenever Janice talked about her experiences at the nudist camps or her home life, it was too stimulating and/or repulsive for her dormitory mates. Some wanted to hear more, while others said it was sick, or sinful. With the slightest encouragement Janice would have continued with nudity whenever convenient for her in the hospital, but the administration was adamant that she could not be allowed to do so. Admittedly Janice would be in the institution a relatively short time and would then return to her family, yet her family's norms were not acceptable and were even attacked by the institution at all levels during her stay there.

There is not only a problem of working out value conflict that might exist between the parents and the institution, the institution has to do the same within. When one considers the large number of significant people in the life of an individual adolescent living in an institution, one needs to appreciate that it is no easy matter for their different life-styles and life values to comfortably mesh. Because sexuality is so disconcerting an area to confront for most people, the difficulties in dealing effectively with sexual issues are compounded. Mayer makes the value conflicts very clear when he describes an institution as having various levels of parenting.[3] (He is not talking about sexuality except perhaps in an implicit fashion.) He describes four levels of parenting — each quite complicated on its own. There is first the level of the "natural parent." Given the complicated life histories of a majority of children living in institutions, this would include not only the biological parents but their various spouses. One might also want to list here the foster parents (often in a succession) with whom the youngster lived prior to placement in the institution. The "child care parent" is the next level and would include not only the direct care staff, who work with the youngster daily, but also the relief staff, recreation staff, housekeeping and maintenance staff — all with whom the child may have important direct interactions. At the next level consider the "therapist parent" or "social worker parent." For a child whose residence in the institution is a lengthy one, there may be many persons at this level. Finally, there is the "authority parent" level where one would include the administration and the consultation staff, whose decisions may also strongly influence the youngster in placement. Contrast this complexity with the "normal family" in its own home in the community where one sees two people who have voluntarily chosen one another and, having committed themselves to a long-term or perhaps permanent relationship, learn to fuse their life-styles.

As regards learning intimacy and values to live by, the adult world may be seen by the adolescent in the institution as being quite fragmented, given the hodgepodge of parent persons. It may never be clear at any moment whose values are prevalent. Also important is that there may not be an immediate model of a caring, committed relationship for the young person to learn from despite the large number of people in charge. It is possible that all of the adults work in the institution and none of them live there. The process whereby these adults work out their differences with one another may not be easily visible. (Disagreements between staff are often not stated in front of the residents so as to not embarass one's colleagues).

Perhaps these may not be considered problematic influences. Rarely do individuals spend a very large number of years of their preadult lives residing in an institution. Adult models have probably been available during the critical earlier years for most. True, these are mitigating circumstances, but they do not fully cancel the importance of an optimal environment during the adolescent years and the cost to the individual who lives in a defective one during this time.

Blos, among others, speaks to the issue of the mutual influence of the adolescent and his/her surroundings.[4] The process is a double one. There are the internal biological hormonal changes of puberty, which can and often do produce personality shifts. There is also the external social environment with its pressures, which also produces personality shifts. Each is an important part of the adolescent developmental process. Greenacre makes the following statement:

> Puberty itself brings new elements of an uneven speed-up of body growth and the appearance of conspicuous changes in body proportions. In addition there are decisive genital developments announcing the physical capacity for full sexual intercourse and parenthood. Menstruation in the girl and the capacity for seminal ejaculations in the boy are so spectacular in themselves as to approach body crises, with inevitable emotional accompaniment in any case. In our culture it is evident that the urgencies of these increased sexual and aggressive drives are generally discrepant with the young person's ability to meet the social and economic responsibilities that would be involved in the fulfillment of implicity demands.[5]

The teenager looks around to see how others deal with these issues. Models are indeed important. They may be real people or aspects of self that one would like to be. The ego ideal is often built on both.

Redl, in talking further about the physiological and feeling changes, cities the earlier research of Bernfeld, which Redl clarifies by somewhat simplifying the nomenclature: the onset of puberty may happen in three entirely different ways. There is the "hesitant" adolescent who reacts to the changes of his or her body and mood with anxiety and even panic. Another type is called the "delinquent" adolescent; here the style is to assume immediately and prematurely all the privileges of adulthood. There is rage at others whenever they attempt to interfere with this. Onset of puberty of the third type Redl calls "manic-depressive." It is a tumultuous pattern with shifts of feelings from deep depressions to crazy wild, omnipotent, delerious feelings.[6] These three patterns of the onset of puberty are greatly affected by the environment in which one lives. For example, in an institution where sexuality is repressed, the "hesitant" adolescent, whose panic reactions to the pubertal shifts are accompanied by much denial of the internal process, gets supportive reinforcement. The "delinquent" adolescent, however, would continually be in difficulty. There needs to be an understanding conveyed to the institutional staff that there are transitional styles of adaptation and that a calming process as well as specific styles of relating to the different patterns needs to be developed. With so many people and each so differently involved, the ongoing, necessary clarification is an extremely complex task.

Unfortunately, this does not complete the list of administrative predicaments. Alas, there is so much more that needs to be said. The ideal of sexual union in our society is a bonding of two people in which the relationship develops with successive small increments of emotional and physical intimacy. These increments become increasingly intertwined so that they finally become interwoven aspects of a unified whole. Examine how the institution fits into this pattern. There is the matter of the constant flow of people into and out of the institution. Youngsters are moved from the community to live for a while in the institution and then moved out perhaps permanently into the community again. Given the large number of persons usually employed at an institution, there are invariably staff leaving to find employment elsewhere and new people coming to work at the institution. Instability of the human environment impedes the task of developing true relational intimacy. While the earliest years of life build the foundations for participating in an intimate relationship as the child develops *object constancy,* adolescence is also a critical time for working on this task.[7]

Not only is the coming and going of people in the lives of the institutional resident a concern in itself, but it is the rare institution that works at teaching what might be involved in entering into and of letting go of a relationship. Sometimes, in fact, the activities of the institution convey the wrong lessons. Note the procedures used to mark the departure of a person from the institution, as described by Trieschman. Often there is a party celebrating the event. Yes, there should be an activity to articulate the loss, but if there is no comcommitant opportunity for appropriate expression of poignant feelings of tender sadness when someone important moves out of our lives, the wrong lesson is conveyed by the party.[8]

Another distortion often taught by institutions has to do with the entry of a new resident into a group. In too many institutions a stranger is brought into intimate living proximity with no opportunity for that person and for the settled residents to explore their feelings about the event (before the placement and for a while after the move). Should we not recognize that this underscores physical proximity as a casual thing?

We need to examine how we teach residents of group living programs to deal with those very painful feelings which come with being rejected. (Who wants to live in an institution?) We do recognize that, in too many cases, the adolescents with whom we work tend to confuse sex with acceptance. In their wish to be lovable, they turn to the warmth of being physically close in the illusion that they are recipients of caring love and all too frequently get hurt again. To show them that they are worthwhile and worth caring for is a major part of their sex education. This is especially important at those times which we might call milestone days, when the individual is reminded by the calendar of the anniversary of his or her entry into the group residence. Birthdays and holidays can also be milestone days. Helping the adolescent to find a way to be in touch with the loneliness and the feelings of being unwanted, yet to not be overwhelmed by these feelings, is the institution's task.

Some institutions for adolescents further complicate the task of mastering sexuality by their residents in not only segregating the resident population according to sex but also by providing only staff of the same gender for the resident group. While this is a problem for children of any age living in group homes, it is particularly poor practice with adolescents. It deprives the teenager of learning basic information about the other sex at a period in life when interest in the other sex is often great, and it also generates a mystique and an intensification of interest in the other sex.

> Fifteen year old Robert was diagnosed as being a youngster with a learning disability. It was not unusual for him to blurt out his thoughts with inappropriate statements. The difficulty in conceptualizing and in organizing his thinking was as familiar to the staff of his residential program as was his poor physical coordination. Since his child care staff were all male, his only real opportunity to have informal interaction with women was at school. The newest teacher was a young women, who was a recent graduate with a degree in special education. Her practice teaching with a population of developmentally disabled children did not adequately prepare her

for Robert's attempts at conversation: "Do you wear a bra?" "How do you know when to kiss?"

While his questions were personal, his wish to know was indicative of a natural adolescent process, blocked by the setting in which he lived. It must be recognized that a residential institution, particularly if it is a large one, is a closed world.

Changing to a coeducational program also may produce problems. It may better prepare the individual resident for relating to the other sex, both during the period of institutional placement and later in life, but it makes the possibility of active heterosexual behavior among the teenagers very likely.

> Artie is an older adolescent who lives in an apartment complex within a larger residential program for retarded boys and girls. The rules concerning physical interaction between the male and female residents are very specific and very restrictive. However, sexuality is not easily erased just because it is officially barred. It goes underground, given the number of residents and the fact of continued available contact between them. Somewhere, somehow, someone manages always to find a way, and others follow. In Artie's institution, the place is the shed behind the administration offices. It is open enough to look innocent but sheltered enough to provide some privacy. That's where Artie lost his virginity, and that's where most of his friends have come for the same purpose.

At some point, it will be discovered by the administration, and access for sexual activities will no longer be possible (at a cost of much staff time, energy, and worry). However, the residents will ultimately locate another place — they always have. Sex finds a way. It may not be as good as the shed, but it will work in its own fashion.

The administration has another option. It can educate its residents about sex. It can teach how to avoid pregnancy and sexually transmitted diseases and otherwise make its staff available to talk over the trials and tribulations of often fickle adolescent sexual attraction and love. The wisdom distilled from the life experience of the staff, and the trust engendered in comfortably talking about feelings, fantasy, and beginning experiences in expressing physical caring in moderate, suitable ways, may be a better control than taboos. But what would the parents of those retarded young people say? What would the community say?

Administrative Concerns

In Artie's institution, sex is altogether forbidden, but of course is does not, cannot go away. The sex moves in another direction rather than stopping altogether. It becomes a group process to a certain extent. Two illustrations follow: (1) Because the shed behind the administration building has almost been entered on several recent occasions by staff at critical points in the sexual experience of some of the residents, they now do not isolate themselves from the group when they go courting. It is no longer an affair of a twosome. They go in small groups ostensibly to play ball, frisbee, or whatever. They are really taking turns at standing guard and courting. There is also some peeking, show and tell, and other attendant activities. (2) Winter storms have made travel hazardous, and the staff coverage is critically low. Supervision of residents is impossible at the previous level. The weather is also too cold for the shed to be useful, so small orgies of kissing, petting, and even intercourse occur in the residences. Because everyone is indoors, these occur in the presence of others. The group is where one lives, eats, and sleeps anyway, so now the group is where sex occurs also.

This is one of the problem features of long-term group living. It tends to blur the separation point between what is private and what is public. Sexual behavior is generally held, in our society, to be a private process involving two people or maybe an individual alone. Group intimate living can influence major modifications in this pattern.

Giallombardo quotes one of her incarcerated delinquent girls: "There is a lot of sex play in the cottages. One girl could be playing with another girl's body. You see it and you ignore it. You're in these surroundings and you look at it every day — kissing and petting and anything else they care to do. You look upon it as an everyday thing. You don't think anything about it."[9]

Not only does the institution have a tendency to distort the development in the individual residents of clarification that will help differentiate the public self from the private self, it is the rare institution that affords adequate privacy to its residents.

There are important reasons from the administrative perspective for maintaining shared living quarters for the resident population in institutions. The costs involved in providing single rooms as compared to room sharing prompt strong considerations for housing residents two or more to a room. Sometimes dormitory or ward sleeping arrangements are used as a way of further reducing costs. Programatically, there are also important considerations for not isolating individuals into solitary rooms. For example, the shy or even the asocial person can benefit from thoughtfully arranged shared housing. Also, where close supervision of residents is important, it can be more easily carried out in a ward rather than with individual sleeping quarters. Whatever the rationale, the result is a lack of privacy. Everyone lives in a fishbowl and there are very few secrets.

One of the most dramatic incidents of this kind involved Norman, fourteen and a half years old, living in a residential treatment institution. He had begun to experiment with variations of masturbation, as is so often the case with many adolescent boys. Norman, however, found himself with a very serious problem that he could not solve by himself. He had made use of a tiny, flexible tube from the gasoline-powered model airplane he was building. The tube was designed to serve as the conduit for gasoline from the container to the tiny airplane engine. Norman had discovered that he could obtain a different sexual effect by inserting it into his penis as though it were a catheter tube, and then masturbating. Unfortunately, he found he could not remove it afterwards. Removal necessitated a trip to the hospital for medical intervention.

What had been a private experience quickly escalated into a public humiliation. Not only were the hospital personnel involved, but the institutional staff at various levels were also given the facts of his dilemma. (An emergency trip to the hospital requires an explanation to fellow staff as to where one is suddenly going, with whom, and why. It requires an explanation of expenses for cab or car, as well as itemization of emergency room and medical fees. The departure of a given child care staff member with one boy unexpectedly also unleashes great curiosity on the part of the other residents, as well as other staff — particularly if a meal time is missed or disrupted.) Unfortunately, not all persons who work in an institution are discreet at all times. Norman's dilemma, sadly, became known to all.

Had a similar experience taken place in a private home, it is not likely that Norman's shame would have been so widely known. In some households even siblings do not learn of each others shameful experiences, due to parental sensitivity and skill. The institution is indeed a community with very few secrets.

Adolescence is a time for experimenting. One finds girls trying different hair styles while boys attempt mustaches and beards. These are some of the outward manifestations of trying to become a sexual person. There is also the need to experiment with non-public parts of one's self. Most institutions discourage this kind of behavior altogether, in very explicit ways. Moreover, the lack of privacy also discourages self-exploration. To the degree that our society in general is not very accepting of these practices, our institutional approach fits the general pattern. There is, however, a difference in that youngsters in their own homes, in greater number than their institutional counterparts, can and do get in touch with their bodies despite the prohibitions. However, the prohibitions take their toll. Masters and Johnson tell us that approximately half the marriages in the United States suffer with some form of sexual dysfunction. There is a strong connection between patterns of self-exploration and self-stimulation and success at other forms of sexual expression later in life.

Dr. Helen Singer Kaplan, who has trained many sex therapists and has written extensively about sexual problems and sexual dysfunctions, feels that sexual ignorance is one of the immediate causes of sexual problems. "The sexual history of a considerable number of dysfunctional couples reveals that they practice poor, insensitive, and ineffective sexual techniques.... In some couples, inadequate lovemaking patterns result from... misinformation and ignorance...."[10]

Lonnie Barbach, in describing her very successful sex therapy program at the University of California Medical Center for helping women attain the fulfillment of their female sexuality, urges self-exploration and self-stimulation as critical steps in the process. "Once you learn about how you respond — through stimulating yourself while free of outside distractions — you will be in a better position to shift your own body movement during love making to achieve more pleasure or to teach your partner how to stimulate you in the manner that is most likely to lead you to sexual pleasure and eventually to orgasm."[11]

There is one other major predicament that faces an administration that would like to build a healthy climate for sexual development of adolescents living in an institution. The problem is one of how to deal with the insidious influence of the resident peer group on one another. The noninstitutionalized adolescent is also greatly influenced by the peer group. However, there are two important dimensions that make for a difference. For the teenager living in a group situation there is no respite or significant escape from the peer group. Its influence is thereby intensified.

The peer group process is omnipresent and always at work. The group norms affect and greatly influence the beliefs and behaviors of the individual. There is no escape from the group precisely because institutions are built on a plan of group living. In contrast to the process in a private home, the activities, conversations, and perceptions are almost invariably geared to the adolescent, rather than adult centered. Polsky describes this very well in his book detailing life in a residential treatment center for adolescents.[12] So telling is the description at times that the reader is ready to come to the mistaken notion that there are no adult caretakers in that program.

This emphasis is particularly marked in regard to sexual attitudes. Regardless of the reason for the institutional placement of each of the resident members, they are a population that can be considered vulnerable. Whether retarded, emotionally disturbed, or physically handicapped, they are not unaware of their special condition. Often they defend themselves from the implications of vulnerability by an overdetermined response that is expressed in a macho attitude (for girls as well as boys) with respect to issues of intimacy and to sexuality in general. All too often this attitude becomes the group norm, continually reinforced in countless ways in the course of daily living.

A vivid portrayal of this feature of institutional living is given by Giallombardo, whose careful research of three separate correctional institutions for girls showed differences in vocabulary but not essentially in inmate culture. It was referred to variously as "the Racket," "the Sillies," and "Chief Business," but in all instances a group sexual norm within the institution prevailed even though it might have been unacceptable for the majority at the times that they might not be institutionalized.[13]

Conclusions

The nature of residential programs for adolescents in the United States is such that major influences intrude on normal sexual development. Consequently, it is difficult, even for a knowledgeable and caring administration, to completely nullify the impact of these intrusions.

There is the matter of privacy. It is the rare institution that affords adequate privacy to its residents. Then there is the extraordinary impact of the adolescent peer group living in the institution. Another complication is that the institution unwittingly stresses a nonrelevance between relational intimacy and physical intimacy. Also, group living makes for beginning patterns of group sex. Not least of all is that there is a continual difference of lifestyle and life values (including sexual values) constantly being aired among the many significant persons who help shape the life of an adolescent living in an institution. The result may be that our institutions produce an altogether different kind of sexual individual than we expect or wish.

REFERENCES

1. Johnson, Joy and Ord Matek. "Critical Issues in Teaching Human Sexuality to graduate Social Work Students," *Journal of Education for Social Work.* vol. 10 no. 3, Fall 1974, pp. 50-55.
   This article describes an approach to this problem with a different kind of group, but the generic aspects of etiology and methods for producing change in the helper group are obvious.
2. Redl, Fritz and David Wineman. *Controls from Within,* The Free Press (Macmillan Co.): New York, 1952, pp. 48-59.
3. Mayer, Morris Fritz. "The Parental Figures in Residential Treatment," *The Social Service Review.* vol. 34 no. 3, September 1960, pp. 273-284.
4. Blos, Peter. *The Adolescent Passage: Developmental Issues.* International University Press: New York, 1978.
5. Greenacre, Phyllis. "Differences Between Male and Female Adolescent Sexual Development as Seen from Longitudinal Studies," in *Adolescent Psychiatry IV.* Feinstein and Giovacchini (eds), Aronson: New York, 1976, p. 108.
6. Redl, Fritz. "Emigration, Immigration and The Imaginary Group" in *Adolescent Psychiatry IV.* Feinstein and Giovacchini (eds), Aronson: New York, 1976, p. 7.
7. Mahler, Margaret, Fred Pine and Anni Bergman. *"The Psychological Birth of the Human Infant,* Basic Books: New York 1975.

8. Trieschman, Albert E. A presentation made at the annual meeting of the American Association for Children's Residential Centers, Chicago, Ill. 1973.
9. Giallombardo, Rose. *The Social World of Imprisoned Girls.* John Wiley and Sons: New York, 1974 p. 244.
10. Kaplan, Helen Singer. *The New Sex Therapy,* Brunner/Mazel: New York, 1974, p. 122.
11. Barbach, Lonnie. *For Yourself: The Fulfillment of Female Sexuality.* Doubleday & Company: Garden City, New York, 1975, Chapter 7.
12. Polsky, Howard. *Cottage Six: The Social System of Delinquent Boys in Residential Treatment.* Russell Sage Foundation: New York, 1962.
13. Giallombardo, Rose. *The Social World of Imprisoned Girls.* John Wiley and Sons: New York, 1974, Chapters 9, 10 and 11.

Chapter Five

LEGAL ISSUES

BURTON JOSEPH AND MARGARET STANDISH

SOCIETY has developed more liberal attitudes toward sexuality in general. The most reliable data reflect an increasing participation, enjoyment, and candor in sexual experiences. Sexuality is celebrated in story and song, in film, the media, and theater.

In spite of this revolution in expression, the moral cloud of our tradition still prohibits, condemns, and criticizes sexual expression among juveniles. The society frowns upon sexual expression and experimation among children, and sexual activity is secretive, suppressed, often guilt ridden, and generally illegal. Although an open society at least offers a potential for sexual activity among adolescents, the social control is absolute in an institutional setting. Adults supervise, monitor, and prohibit the open expression of sexuality. The attitude of repression that is prevalent can be fully implemented in an institutional environment.

The law prohibits sexual activity between juveniles (defined by different ages in different jurisdictions) so that even outside of institutions, by legal definition, all sexual activity must either be masturbatory or elicit. The law does not recognize such a thing as a healthy, rewarding, satisfying sexual experience for a child. Even sexual activity that is tolerated, but by no means encouraged, such as kissing, petting, and holding hands, is denied in institutional settings by the force of authority.

Administrative efforts to reduce sexual contact are a reflection of prevailing moral and legal attitudes as well as a design for the convenience of the administration in running the institution. It is often justified as protection of exploitation of the juveniles confined; indeed, that is frequently the case. The legal rational is that sexual relations among juveniles cannot be "voluntary" because juveniles (usually under the age of 18) cannot legally "consent." Coercion, then is more a definition of law than it is a statement of fact.

The law and its handmaiden — traditional attitudes toward sexuality — encourage this control and create an inevitable conflict between natural sexual curiosity and development on one hand and legislative and moral constraints upon sexual activity on the other.

Normal relationships between children and adults, children and children, and children and the world outside are perverted in an institutional setting. The law treats sexual needs of juveniles in confinement as if such needs do not exist.

The problem is exacerbated by traditional and virtually universal segregation by sex in institutions. Sex education and dissemination of useful information are virtually nonexistent. Contraception, which may be difficult to obtain outside of the institution, is totally unavailable within. The laws of some states that prohibit dispensation of contraceptive information and devices can be totally enforced within the institution. Ignorance pervades in matters of sexually transmitted diseases and reproduction. If laws or policies exist against the teaching of sexuality in the community in general, they find total fulfillment in the atmosphere of confinement.

Masturbation seems to remain the only outlet, which must be done surreptitiously or with homosexual mutuality. Even assuming privacy is available for personal fantasies, there is the omnipresent guilt, fear of exposure, and participation in ways that may be contrary to the individual's sexual orientation.

Under a recent decision of the United States Supreme Court, parents can commit juveniles as "voluntary" patients in a mental institution, regardless of how vigorously the child objects. Absolute control in terms of parental discretion for confinement or treatment is sanctioned by the law. Independent inquiry from the child's perspective is not afforded as a matter of right, and no procedures are required once such "voluntary" hospitalization is commenced. Although this is most often a result of good will and for admirable objectives on behalf of parents, guardians, and attending medical personnel, the dicisions are frequently made from the psychological and social orientation of a different generation. Abuses, although relatively infrequent, are well documented. Liberty, then, for an adolescent can be denied through mental commitment at the request of a parent or guardian.

In the judicial process, as distinct from therapeutic hospitalization, due process of law frequently affords some although only minimal protection for juveniles. The laws to declare a child delinquent, dependant, or a minor in need of supervision vary from state to state but universally fall short of what is considered due process in adult terms. Confinement by judicial decree for acts that do not constitute violations of any law are frequent; these so-called "status offenses" deprive juveniles of their liberty, often on such petty grounds as disobedience, truancy, running away (even though it is recognized that the child who flees is often the healthiest member of the family unit), or insubordination.

Even minor criminal offenses, such as shoplifting and pot smoking, can result in long periods of detention when the same act, if committed by an adult processed through the legal system, would result in a small fine or at most a few days in a local jail. The accepted procedure is to permit detention up to and even after the ward becomes an adult so long as the alleged offense was committed as a juvenile. As the United States Supreme Court has pointed out, the child is often left with a loss of liberty, a denial of due process, and no counseling, treatment, educational opportunity, or recreational facilities. It is the worst of both worlds. During confinement the denial of sexual expression that might otherwise by available becomes absolute.

The loss of privacy during institutionalization and the susceptibility and frequency of sexual abuse by older, stronger, and more street wise inmates perverts normal sexual development. This result, ironically, is justified as being in the best interest of the child.

Initial sexual contacts will invariably be homosexual and often accompanied by force under totally asexual or antisexual circumstances and for domination and control rather than for sexual fulfillment. This occurs under the sanction of law during a most impressionable period of sexual development.

These problems never come to the attention of courts for several reasons. The most obvious reason is that there are no legal rights of minors with regard to sexual matters. Since there are no rights, there is no basis for seeking any judicial relief. A search of legal precedent fails to reveal a single incident where the sexual needs or rights of children have ever been recognized or considered, let alone enforced. Even if such a right did exist, where would the child in an institution find the human and financial resources to seek legal redress? Certainly not from the administrators or counselors; certainly not from law enforcement officials; certainly not from the parents or guardians.

Even if all of these burdens were overcome, it is highly unlikely that any relief would be granted because the courts, following the lead of the United States Supreme Court, are extremely reluctant to interfere with administrative discretion in running an institution of confinement. It is certainly ironic that sexual promiscuity is a recognized basis for institutionalizing juveniles — especially young women — and that the punishment is not only restriction of liberty but deprivation of any semblance of normal sexual contact.

ABORTION

The Supreme Court has ruled that abortion is a matter of privacy between patient and physician and is a right protected by the Constitution of the United States. Efforts to restrict abortions, at least during the first trimester of pregnancy, are prohibited. Thereafter, reasonable restrictions relating to the health and welfare might be appropriate, but the right to abortion cannot be denied. Subsequent decisions have affirmed that this is a right enjoyed not only by adult women but also by minors, and efforts to intervene between the minor patient and her physician so as to deny or restrict abortion have generally been stricken as unconstitutional. The courts have so far recognized that the choice to terminate a pregnancy is to be made between the minor and her physician and is not subject to veto by parents or benevolent administrators.

The problems of abortion are exacerbated, of course, in an institutional setting. Access to information, alternatives, or advice on a true physician/patient basis is severely restricted. The juvenile, while enjoying a legal right, is under severe stress by virtue of the institutional setting and much more amenable to official decision on her behalf. Involuntary abortions remain unconstitutional and illegal, but threats and coercion are not unheard of, which result in the dubious granting of consent. In addition, just because a legal right exists does not suggest that the means are available to assert or to take advantage of its benefits. A pregnant adolescent in an institution must still find an understanding physician, arrange for the procedure, and have the resources to seek legal redress if the right is denied. An opportunity to be heard or counseled by a sympathetic adult responsible for arrangements and implementation of her legal right may not be available. One can speculate on the converse situation also, where an adolescent wishes to continue her pregnancy but is under severe pressure from institutional administrators or parents or guardians to terminate her pregnancy. How rare the juvenile who could resist the inherently coersive circumstances that institutionalization creates and exercise an independent will. No studies could be found that address this problem, and the conclusion is speculative; however, the pervasive attitude in juvenile institutions that "poppa knows best" very likely extends to this area of sexual privacy as well as others.

CONCLUSION

The courts and institutions do not recognize that a legal problem exists regarding the sexuality of adolescents in institutions. No court decision, law review article, or commentary could be found that addresses the rights, needs, or the fulfillment of adolescent sexuality in an institutional setting. It is not so much that a problem does exist but that it is not recognized or considered.

Chapter Six

SEX EDUCATION PROGRAMS FOR RESIDENTS

Jean Schaar Gochros

DESPITE our supposed sexual liberation, the area of sex education is fraught with anxiety and tension. Even generally knowledgeable and enthusiastic supporters, whether parents, teachers, staff members, administrators, or "helping" professionals, can become overwhelmed with self-doubt and uncertainty when faced with probems of deciding who should be taught what, where, when, how, by whom, and with what degree of knowledge. When the proposed program is for adolescents whose institutionalization has automatically defined them as special or different from the rest of the population, anxiety increases.

Such anxiety often leads people in predictable directions. Some may insist that sex education is not the institution's responsibility. Indeed, many people question whether the institutionalized have sexual rights; others deny or ignore their needs while going to great lengths to try to prevent them from even "getting any ideas," much less expressing their sexuality. At the other extreme, institutional staff jump blindly into a formal program with inadequate planning, retreating when the program is met with resistance or runs into unanticipated problems (as it invariably does). Others may provide a few facts and conclude that the job is done. A common approach is a frantic search and demand for curriculum cookbooks with fail-safe recipes. When none are found, the decision is made to abandon sex education rather than risk error, which is often equated with failure.

Trying to provide such cookbooks is futile. The anxiety about sex education stems not from a lack of recipes but from a variety of contradictory myths, misconceptions, and rules about sex and sex education. It is often more helpful to start by taking time to recognize these myths and rules and their effect on us, to provide ourselves with more freeing concepts, and to examine ideas about how to put those concepts to use.

This chapter will attempt to do just that; it will start with the myths and replace them with a concept of "planned" sex education that can be used for any person of any age in any setting. It will then translate those concepts into an institutional setting, suggesting some considerations that must be part of program planning. Finally, it will suggest both unique aspects and unifying themes to consider in sifting through the specific needs of a specific institution.

Myths, Misconceptions, and Contradictory Rules

Our first problem in sex education is that we live in a transition period tied to the myths, misinformation, and dictums of the reproductive bias, overlaid with contradictory myths and dictums of today. Concepts that are truly liberating are still evolving, and there is, of course, a wide range of values that people hold regarding sexuality. Of course, many — perhaps most — people still struggle without realizing it, caught in the conflict between old and new ideas. This same struggle is reflected in a myriad of equally confusing and contradictory ideas about sex education, which again affect us without our even being aware of their existance. Consider just a few of these ideas:

(1) Sex education is a course like (and about) biology, giving a few facts and values about reproduction, menstruation, V.D., intercourse, and pregnancy. (2) Since very few people should be having babies, very few have sexual needs, and very few should be given this course. (3) They do not need this course until they are ready to make babies. (4) We can decide to whom we will give this course, when and where it will be given, when it will stop, what we will give, who will teach it, and what our students will learn. (5) Those who are not given it will not learn about sex. (6) We do not need to learn about sex, because sex is so instinctive that we all know all about it. (7) We need no knowledge to teach it, for the same reason. (8) On the other hand, sex educators must know everything there is to

know about it (especially biology), and need know nothing more than biology. (9) All sex educators should agree, and should have perfect sex lives themselves. (10) We can give sex education without ever talking about sex. (11) We are only giving it when we are talking about it. (12) We should give values but not facts; on the other hand, we should give facts but not values. (13) Our students will learn what we tell them, act on it immediately, and remember it forever. (14) Adults are totally responsible for what children learn and do; if a child gets in trouble, the adult is to blame. (15) Adults have no responsibility; if the child gets into trouble, it is entirely his or her fault.

Finally — the cardinal rules of our modern "liberated" sex education:

> Always answer a child's questions, but never answer unless asked; never provide more than is asked, but *always be warm, relaxed, totally comfortable, and totally honest.*

It is little wonder that so many people are terribly anxious about sex education. They have set impossible goals for themselves. They fear that if they err for a moment in their facts, values, emotions, or even in unintended clues about their own imperfect sex lives, they will either create irreparable emotional scars or corrupt innocent young minds. They are sure they will be failures as parents, professionals, and even responsible citizens; they are equally sure that there is a right way to provide sex education, if only some expert will tell them how.

A New Look at Sexuality and Sex Education

Let's push aside our old, rigid concepts and make way for new and less rigid ones. Freed from the confines of the reproductive bias, sex education can encompass not only subjects such as intercourse and reproduction but a complex totality of ideas, emotions, functions, and processes that interweave and defy brief, rigid definitions. For example, it can include our ideas of masculinity and feminity and our expectations for each gender; social and interpersonal skills necessary for different kinds of relationships; and our ideas about warmth, affection, and intimacy. It can futher include physiological responses that may vary according to the person, the moment, the situation — even according to one's cultural beliefs. It includes imagination and fantasy. If we think of sex in terms of sensuality (the giving and receiving of pleasure via the body), allowing for the pleasurable aspects of sex as well as the work (reproductive) aspects, we open up a whole new range of options from thumbsucking, cuddling, caressing, and backrubbing to self-stimulation, genital caressing to orgasm, oral sex, and intercourse. Thus sex education is about activities that may or may not lead to orgasm, may or may not include intercourse, may or may not require a person of the other gender or another person at all. They may not even require any part of the body besides a brain. Indeed, some totally paralyzed people report having pleasurable imaginary orgasms.

Such a view of sexuality immediately lessens anxiety for both the professional and the student/client. This is particularly true for those who were heretofore excluded purely because of their age and their institutionalization. It recognizes the need, capability, and right of *everyone* to enjoy some form of sexuality from birth to death. It does require several rules for responsibility and morality:

> After infancy, we are responsible to some degree for the consequences of our actions. In sex, as in other areas, we should treat ourselves and others with dignity and respect. We should try to maximize emotional and physical pleasure while inflicting minimal emotional and physical pain. We should respect our own and others' (including the potential "others" who have not yet been conceived or born) needs, capabilities, rights, and wishes. We should respect any given culture's codes of public conduct.

Such a broad generalization lessens anxiety about value giving, for it allows each person to determine his or her own options and code of morality without interfering with the rights of others. It demands responsibility but allows everyone to take that responsibility at his or her own level of ability.

It takes away the mysterious, exclusive ideas of sex education by redefining it as the giving and receiving of facts and values about sexuality through a socialization process in which we are all students and teachers continually, from birth to death. The messages we receive and give are formal and informal, planned and unplanned, subtle and explicit, conscious and unconscious. They are given in every conceivable way using all of our senses. They are transmitted by actions and words, as well as by lack of action and words.

Our "educators" are ourselves, our parents, physicians, teachers, nurses, playmates, ministers, babysitters, classmates, neighbors, people sitting next to us in movies, etc. Also, let us not forget the entire range of media events that bombard us continually. The explicit messages are sometimes less effective than the implicit ones we receive unconsciously, but they are potentially more useful, since they are subject to monitoring, deliberate reinforcement or negation, and hopefully, rational evaluation.

Most of this education is unplanned. It cannot be prevented by parents, teachers, professionals, or administrators. Those adults who choose not to say anything about sex will nevertheless be giving sex education. Whether this education is helpful or harmful will be strictly up to chance. Since it is often spontaneous gut reaction, it may not be congruent with what the teacher would like to have imparted, and it gives little chance for either the receiver or other responsible adults to provide thoughtful evaluation. Hence, the most useful education is that which maximizes both the amount of planned messages and the degree of congruence between planned and unplanned messages.

Planned Sex Education

Planned sex education is derived from the following: (1) recognition that we are all unplanned sex educators whether we wish to be or not; (2) a decision about how much responsibility we ourselves will take for providing education and how much we will ask others to take; (3) a reasonable amount of knowledge and advance thought about our attitudes toward various sexual behaviors, sex roles, lifestyles, etc. (4) a considerable effort to make our unplanned messages congruent with our planned education.

In other words, it is a deliberate attempt to provide access to whatever new ideas, skills, knowledge, and resources are necessary for people to find responsible sexual fulfillment in accordance with their needs and abilities. To accomplish this task, one must be willing to —

1. Make a reasonable attempt to examine one's own knowledge and attitudes, enhance knowledge, and then reevaluate one's attitudes in the light of new knowledge;
2. Have courage to state one's own convictions, the honesty to admit that they may not be shared by others and may

not even be right, and the willingness to allow and encourage others to state theirs;
3. Have courage to share feelings, admit gaps in knowledge and errors, and the willingness to cooperate with others in correcting errors and filling in the gaps;
4. Anticipate and rehearse the questions, situations, and probblems that might arise and how one might deal with them;
5. Recognize that headaches are a part of life;
6. Keep a supply of aspirin, imagination, and humor on hand.

Thus, we use anything (objects, words, actions, events) to either directly or indirectly help people gain the knowledge, comfort, skill, and resources necessary for responsible sexual fulfillment. By using our own creativity, we have an abundance of techniques at our disposal, and a myriad of co-teachers. We can turn the whole world and anything in it into more useful door openers. We can give unplanned socialization techniques purpose and meaning and turn errors into enlightening opportunities. Our planned sex education program can include planned reactions and nonreactions, one liners, informal conversations, semiformal rap sessions, and formalized courses with lectures. Following are examples, some verbal, some written, some actions:

"Say, I was just thinking. You're really growing up. Maybe you'd like to know how your body is going to start changing."

"Wow! That's a hard question to answer. Let me think about it for a minute."

"See this box? It has something only for women, because something happens to women each month. When it starts happening to them, they know they're really growing up. Let me explain what happens, and let's start showing you how to use these pads."

"It's fine if you want to feel your penis – I know it feels good. But you should do it in private."

"This TV program is good. C'mon in and watch it with me."

"I hear your school started classes on sex last week. Why don't we talk a bit about how it's going and what you think of it. And maybe we can talk about some of the questions that schools sometimes forget to answer."

Door openers serve many functions. Some provide information, some express attitudes or rules, and some are a combination.

All door openers, however, have certain things in common. They capitalize on starting where the person is, on respecting difference, and on accepting error. They use such communication techniques as open-ended questions, "many people" or "everybody" starters, and include warmth, empathy, and honesty. They implicitly allow for humor, lending themselves to such techniques as "looseners" for formal sessions. For example:

> "Well, here we are in a class designed to make us feel comfortable about sex, and we're all uncomfortable as hell. I wonder why. Bet we can find out. Remember the first time you asked how babies are made? What answer did you get?"
>
> Have a group shout out all the sexual words they can think of, especially the forbidden ones.

It usually takes little time for the group to release tension through laughter and to start spontaneous, useful discussion.

True, in some ways we are asking people to take more responsibility but it is a tenable, freeing responsibility because it legitimates disagreement, error, and discomfort. The special beauty of this approach is that it can be easily modified to fit the needs of any person, situation, or setting, and can be initiated whenever one wishes. Hence, it is appropriate for any institution and reduces the number of unique probelms to a more manageable number.

Meanwhile, Back at the Insitution

Spouting a few pearls of wisdom and giving a few one-liner examples is easy. The real work starts when the time comes to translate general ideas into a real life program. While no chapter or book can make that final translation for you, it is possible to give some guidelines that will help. The next few pages will revisit the basic ingredients of planned sex education: (1) advance thought or planning; (2) anticipation and rehearsal; and (3) door openers.

These concepts will be explored as they relate to program planning. Keep in mind two facts: (1) *Program* is loosely defined here as encompassing a broad approach from informal door openers to very formal courses; and (2) *Planning* is a total and continual process. The three aspects of planned sex education do not always occur sequentially, but in a continual cycle with considerable overlapping.

Advance Thought

Advance thought or program planning is a shared responsibility, starting with you. Hence, you must address the following questions: What are your concerns? Why do you want a program? What is your place in the institution? What are your knowledge base and your attitudes about masturbation, oral sex, homosexuality, contraception and abortion, sexually transmitted disease, and premarital or extramarital sex? What are your responsibilities, and who shares your concerns? What is the line of authority in your institution, and will you need to start from the bottom up, the top down, or across your peer circle in initiating a sex education program?

Expanding Knowledge and Value Base. Once you have thought about these core questions you will need to rethink them with others. As your unit or total staff begins to share knowledge and values, you will have to decide where there are areas of agreement and disagreement, what are the highest and lowest levels of expertise in your midst, and what is the basic minimum needed by each. You may find that your next step needs to be some formal in-service training. What are the resources for such training? Can you yourself provide it? Can your unit? What about having the staff enroll in a continuing education workshop? Can a community expert be hired to bring a workshop to the institution? Do you have a consultant already available to assist in training and program planning?

What is the Institution Structure and Population, and What Kind of Program Does it Need? In our definition of planned sex education, there are several options for the kind of program that is needed, dependent upon the structure of your institution and the population it serves. Are you a small group home for just a few children? Is your staff small and do your adolescents attend a public school that already has a sex education program? Then maybe the only "formal" sessions you will need will be for staff, and the "program" will consist of the same door openers that any family uses in everyday conversations and heart-to-heart talks. Is it a large institution with a school of its own? Then you may want a formal program within that school, a semiformal program of discussion sessions, an informal but planned program of conversational door openers to supplement the formal program or a combination of all of these.

No matter what, you will need to decide who is responsible for the program and what the nature of that responsibility will be. Will it be one person doing all the formal teaching and planning? Will it be one unit or a social work or psychology department? Will it be an overall program in which each teacher, department, or houseparent is given the general framework or topic for the day and handles it with his or her own charges in semiautonomous fashion? Will it be an overall program in which each staff member operates almost autonomously? Or perhaps, in a small unit such as a ward of chronically ill or dying teenagers in a hospital, will it be periodic discussion sessions that include all staff members?

Remember that no matter what the program, there will be unplanned sex education going on. A truly planned approach will try to integrate the planned and unplanned through periodic staff meetings to assess the situation, coordinate efforts, and discuss problems. Ideally, there should be at least one person responsible for the total program (although he or she may delegate particular duties), for twenty or thirty cooks each acting autonomously may create more confusion than help. That person may act as teacher, coordinator, consultant, trainer, trouble shooter, liason person to administrators, families, or to the public at large. The extent to which he or she assumes or delegates responsibility will again depend on the structure of the institution and the individual's job description. If sex education is merely one of many duties, for instance, it will be unrealistic to assume responsibility for everything, and coordination may be the only function. The responsibility for the total program is a difficult one, for the biggest problems often come not from the residents but from problems within the staff; such as personality clashes, differences in style and values, and problems of professional turf. Hence, attention must be paid to the expertise of that leader, the nature of leadership and the authority he or she is accorded.

Who Is the Leader? The leader should have at least some degree of professional training in sexuality and sex education within the helping professions. One should remember that medical, religious, or psychiatric training does not insure knowledge about sexuality or skill in working with people in such programs, nor does the existence of emotional or physical illness in people necessarily alter the basic content they need in sex education. No matter who is the leader is, he or she will have areas of both strength and weakness and will need to call on others' expertise, as well as have the ability to work with people from various professions.

Authority. The myths mentioned earlier give rise to some unique problems in sex education. One is that while people are often loathe to recognize their own expertise and assume responsibility for leadership, the person who does so is immediately surrounded by colleagues who are suddenly far more expert, wise, and sensitive than the leader. That person will need to use tact and sensitivity in dealing with colleagues, but he or she will be helpless unless backed by official recognition and accorded power. For that reason, it is often helpful to hire an outsider to take the job. If using an expert from outside means that expertise from inside has been overlooked, however, the resulting resentment will be both justified and damaging.

The Nature of Leadership. Just as tact without authority is meaningless, so is authority without tact; the two are inseparably bound. Whether leadership responsibility is given to one person or a team, the leader must use both authority and sensitivity to create a delicate balance. Leadership should be enabling without being authoritarian; it must share knowledge, but that sharing should include honesty, humor, and comfort about one's own errors. The group must be a support group that offers honest critique, advice, and help to its members without competition and destructive criticism.

Allowance must be made for differences in values and styles, and ways must be found to help adolescents deal with difference, without undermining staff members or throwing the adolescent into undue turmoil. Yet starting a sex education program is no different from starting any other program that calls for new methods, values, or techniques. While every attempt must be made to engage resistant staff, there must be a base level of expectations and standards, adherence to ground rules, and integrity.

Anticipation and Rehearsal

Any program, no matter how informal it may be, should contain provision for continual anticipation of problems, rehearsal, feedback, and reevaluation. This may mean planned time both prior to and following formal class or discussion sessions, or periodic meetings at reasonably close intervals for strictly informal programs. Of course, not all feedback and rehearsal need to be formal, but unless there is time set aside for it, the support system needed to make a truly planned educational program will soon be lost. It is through these sessions that the real art, skill, and comfort about sex education may be gained, provided that this time is used to deal with issues and ideas, to ask for and receive help, and to truly rehearse potentially or proven difficult scenes. Rehearsal through role playing is often far more useful than purely intellectual discussion. The following scenario with a team of house-parents, social workers, and psychologists in a treatment institution for emotionally disturbed adolescents may serve as an example:

Ted: I need help. Joey is still worrying about masturbation and asked me yesterday if I ever do it. I think I goofed. I told him I couldn't answer him because what people do sexually is a private matter.

Lynn: Well, you just gave him our ground rule about asking personal questions. That doesn't sound do bad.

John: Yeah. What's the problem? Are you upset about masturbation?

Ted: No — it's fine with me. But I don't want him to think he has to do it just because I do it, any more than I want him to feel guilty about it just because his father gets so upset.

Sue: True. And if he thinks it's so evil, how will he feel about you? And might he get caught in conflict between you and his father?

Ted: That's what I was concerned about. But I think I upset him even more this way. I need ideas on how to deal with this in the future, and how to help Joey now. Can we role play it? I thought of one possibility I want to try out.

Three or four plays follow, with different people trying out their ideas. Each is critiqued for strengths and weaknesses, but no one is truly satisfied with the options.

Leader: You know, it strikes me that none of us are willing to just answer Joey honestly. Are we copping out? Is our ground rule so sacred and would we really be giving away secrets? Or are we just assuming Joey will be upset by reality because he has a label "emotionally disturbed." How can he deal with reality if nobody tells him what reality is? Ted, let me try a different approach with you.

Ted: Okay. (Role playing Joey's part). Do you ever masturbate?

Leader: Oh, well sure! Almost everybody does, including most adults, even those who believe it's wrong and try their best not to do it.

John: Right! What's important, Joey, is not what your Dad or I or other people do, but that we help you decide what *you* think about it, and when it's okay or not okay for *you*.

Ted: Okay, that does it for me! I'd feel comfortable with that combination, and I know how to take it from there. I think it would help all the kids and reinforce what I say to Joey, though, if Sue and John talk about masturbation in their Sunday rap session.

Lynn: I agree. Leader, I have one more question. What do we do if Joey starts asking whether we have oral sex?

Leader: (Looking at watch) You say quickly, "Time's-up-go-ask-your father."

Everyone laughs. John thinks it can be dealt with in the same way; the others disagree. The decision is made that this will be discussed during the next meeting.

Parent Involvement

Although it is not always practical or possible to do so, particularly in residential facilities, the more parents can be involved in the teenager's planned sex education, the more useful the program will be. This means making every attempt to engage the parent as a team member in shared responsibility, using the same door openers that one uses with either the residents or colleagues. This may include parent-staff workshops, phone calls, or short notes to alert either the staff or the family to a particular problem or to give feedback, or merely a brief discussion of sexuality included in a general discussion with a parent about a child's progress.

Ground rules must be set that will protect confidentiality, yet will allow for parental and staff intervention in a problem when necessary. Again there must be planning to work out ways of handling disagreement, to reinforce agreed-on values, to share knowledge, and offer mutual help.

Course Content

General topics have already been suggested, applicable to any type of program. More specific curriculum guides for formal courses are available. However, these guidelines should not be used as rigid "recipes." With all of the problems an institutional program may present, there may be one real advantage: the planners can be far more creative and flexible than they might be in a set school system and can individualize the program to fit the students' needs at any given point.

Door openers are especially pertinent here, for a course or program may be far more useful and more easily accepted if tied to events or issues of immediate concern to the students. For example, in a home for unwed mothers, the starting point may be issues of birth control or pregnancy. In a correctional institution, the door opener may be general problems or a specific instance of homosexual rape. In a medical setting, the door opener may be how a particular illness affects sexuality. In an institution in which adolescents often take charge of smaller children, the subject might best be introduced in a discussion of how to deal with the sexual behaviors and questions of young children.

Humor

Many people approach sex so soberly that it reinforces rather than negates the frightening mystique surrounding it. Humor is just as appropriate in sex education as it is anywhere else. As long as an attitude of snickering is avoided, and as long as it is true humor rather than ridicule at the expense of another person, humor can be your strongest ally, relieving tension while giving perspective to the place of sexuality in one's life.

Individualizing to Fit the Needs of Specific Institutions

While this chapter can hardly deal with the specific needs of a variety of institutions, it is obvious that a program for one setting will face different problems and may need to be far different from a program in another setting. For example, a program for the retarded will need to take into account special problems in learning and teaching without being intimidated by myths that the retarded cannot learn or that they have different sexual needs and abilities from others. This means that all the problems found and solutions used in work with others will be exaggerated in an institution for the retarded. Door openers will be needed more often, not less. Information, values, and social skills will need to be taught more concretely, simply, and creatively. Rules for public conduct will need to be given and repeated, with attention to specific circumstances. The problems of adults may need to be given in terms that small children can understand. Repetition and feedback will be especially important, as will individualization according to needs and abilities.

A program in a correctional facility may have to focus more on problems of authority, power, and coercion and will have to face the realities of a harsh punitive system without being defeated by those realities. This means that the adolescents may need special help in dealing with concerns about homosexuality, maintaining self-esteem, facing oppression without perpetuating it, and differentiating between the values of a prison population and the values of the larger society. There may be special skills, knowledge, and creativity needed to deal effectively with staff differences, cultural differences (or stereotypes), and intense peer pressures.

Unifying Themes

No matter what the specifics of the institution, programs may be individualized with basic unifying themes. All residents will need both self-respect and respect from others. All will be struggling with problems of self-identity, loneliness, and a sense of isolation and difference. All will want love but will risk vulnerability only to the extent that they can be reasonably sure they will not be physically or emotionally hurt. All will need help in realistically facing their handicap (whether it is an intellectual, emotional, physical, or social one) and in planning around it while maintaining self-esteem.

Despite behavioral problems that may have either caused or been created by institutionalization, the basic sexual needs and concerns of adolescents in institutions are no different from those of other adolescents. No matter what the program, that is the basic message that must be imparted. Furthermore, the adolescent must know that he or she has the right to responsible sexual expression. To pay lip service to that right, however, without doing anything to provide true access to responsible sexual expression is not enough. It is of little value, for instance, to tell the retarded to conduct their sexual activities in private if the institution makes no provision for privacy. One would hope that sex education would include values about affection, respect, and dignity, but it would be sheer insanity to expect an adolescent inmate to deal with rapists by insisting that they treat her or him with more respect. Sex educators will need to be realistic and honest about both the deliberate and the unintentional sexual oppression that the institutionalized adolescent faces. At the same time, they must offer any assistance possible in eradicating or at least alleviating such oppression.

In summary, when dealing with sex, we are talking about an integral part of human life. Sex education, then, is not merely a course about biology and genitalia. It is a program for dealing with life, in which the institution must take responsibility for helping to make that life as free of pain and full of joy as is humanly possible.

Chapter Seven

IN-SERVICE TRAINING PROGRAMS FOR STAFF

O. Dale Kunkel

Introduction

ADMINISTRATORS of residential training programs for adolescents must deal on a daily basis with the problems of promoting normal sexual development in what amounts to an abnormal environment. Given that adolescence is a period of sexual turmoil under the best of circumstances, the reconciliation of the sexual/developmental needs of adolescents with the mechanistic requirements of the institutional bureaucracy is among the most perplexing of the administrator's tasks.

In-service training on the subject of sexuality is frequently one of the first strategies employed in trying to reconcile the sexual needs of adolescents with the exigencies of the institutional environment. The choice of training as an administrative strategy is not surprising, since we in this country have a historical preference for educational solutions to social problems. It is important to recognize, however, that staff training is not a panacea. There are unique problems involved in sexual training, and these problems are not infrequently exacerbated by the incongruities between sexual needs and institutional realities. In fact, on more than one occasion sex education has generated more problems than it has solved. We shall explore some of the reasons why this is true in the course of this chapter.

The purpose of this chapter is to outline the major issues in developing a staff training program in sexuality, to point out some common pitfalls, to suggest major topics to be considered in designing the program, and finally to offer a conceptual format within which staff training and development may be seen as a comprehensive and ongoing process.

Considerations in Staff Development Planning

There are several factors that need to be borne in mind in designing staff development programs on sexuality. Underscoring each of these factors will be a consistent caveat: *beware of prepackaged training programs that fail to take into account the individual needs and circumstances of a particular institution*. The needs of adolescent residential institutions vis-a-vis sexuality are unique and complex, and a careful assessment is necessary. The time and effort expended in needs assessment and planning will be more than repaid, while the apparent convenience of prepackaged training programs will often result in lost staff time and little in the way of performance improvement.

With the foregoing as warning, what are the factors that need to be considered in the training needs of staff residents? Several will be discussed.

The Reason the Adolescent is Institutionalized. We might regard this as the presenting problem that has led to the adolescent being in the residential institution. Most adolescents in such a setting have experienced serious developmental or behavioral problems. Factors such as physical illness or handicap, emotional disturbance, family breakdown, or mental retardation may be the reason the adolescent has been placed in a residential facility. Each of these problem constellations may have serious implications for the sexual development of the teenager. Not infrequently, sexual behavior itself may be part of the reason that the adolescent is in the institution. In our culture, this is particularly true for females (Wooden, 1976). Whether the reasons for institutionalization directly or indirectly involve sexuality, they have a direct bearing on the planning of staff development programs.

The Nature of the Institution. Since we are concerned here with sexuality in an institutional context, we are *ipso facto* not talking about normal adolescent sexuality (whatever that is). Institutions often have a pathogenic effect on behavior, and sexuality is frequently one of the first victims of the institutional environment (Hirayama, 1979). While institutions (as we are using that term) vary widely in structure and operation, they all share to some extent in the tendency to regulate resident's behavior according to formal rules, to depersonalize residents, to restrict individual choices, and to deny residents responsibility for their own behavior (Goffman, 1961). Each of these institutional traits may pose problems in promoting functional sexual adjustment and behavior for the residents.

The Social Mandates and Limits of Institutions. Most residential institutions for adolescents operate *in loco parentis* but do not have at their disposal the same range of options that society and circumstances grant to natural parents. The limits on institutions are both formal and informal in nature. Informally, many parents are vague, ambivalent, and even hypocritical in their handling of adolescent sexuality (Chilman, 1977). In general, they know that their adolescent children must grow and experiment with their emerging sexuality, but they often do not want to know *too* much about precise activities. The parental tendency to look the other way is an option not always open to formal social service agencies. Most agencies are much more open to public scrutiny and criticism than are families. The need exists, therefore, to develop formal policies on many issues that families treat with indirection and ambivalence.

That most institutions have multiple caretakers poses yet another problem. The legitimacy of caretakers imposing their own sexual standards on residents is questionable and is another pressure on the institutions to develop consistent rules and policies on sexual conduct. The alternative is to expose the residents to a potpourri of opinions and expectations from different staff persons. In trying to formulate clear and practical rules, the administrator may be forced to deal with many issues that heretofore have submerged in relation to resident's sexual needs and behaviors.

The Standards and Expectations of the Community. Since social agencies are subject to public scrutiny and act as agents for the community, there is a frequent pressure for them to be beyond reproach. The agency must formulate clear and defensible policies, and inevitably these will conflict with the standards of some segment of the community. In addition, larger agencies with non-professional and paraprofessional staff must be aware that the staff members come into the agencies as bearers of community norms. A training program that fails to take account of these sources of community influence may quickly run aground. This is not to say that the agency should slavishly adhere to the mores of the community. Qualified agencies have the opportunity, and indeed the responsibility, to provide leadership to the community in this area. However, the vagaries of community expectations are one more reason to beware of the training package approach.

The Dynamics of Adolescent Adjustment. Adolescence is a time of often painful transition, uncertainty, exploration, and limit testing. Sexuality is a major theme of adolescent development and a frequent point of rebellious reaction against parental (or parental surrogate) influence. The need of the formal institution for rules and policies should never be allowed to obscure the need for compassion and responsiveness to the needs of particular individuals. A basic value premise in this chapter is that we should design training programs (in fact, the entire ethos of the institution) to encourage self-discovery rather than compliance. Toward this end, the final section of this chapter will discuss some measures by which it may be possible to overcome the structural limitations of the agency and perhaps even turn them to the mutual advantage of the institution and the residents.

Common Errors in Sex Education

The Sex Information and Education Council of the United States has identified four common errors that afflict sex education programs. These errors provide a useful point of departure for our consideration.

Sex education versus "reproduction" education — this refers to the familiar tendency to confine sex education programs to relatively safe topics such as sexual anatomy. This so-called "plumbing" emphasis neglects other vital social and emotional aspects of sex which are of frequent concern to adolescents.

Sex education as something given — this refers to a common bias which is evident in the techniques of sex education. Often an "authority" imparts his/her wisdom about sexuality, without opportunity for reaction or interaction. This approach ignores the necessity of self-exploration and interpersonal exchange. The effect is to minimize the integration of the material presented.

Sex education as insurance against moral disaster — this approach places emphasis on the information which will keep the learner "out of trouble." It tends to offer a single viewpoint, minimizes different perspectives, and ignores the fact that sexuality is more than just a source of danger. It often advances a narrow value code which is inherently afraid of sex. Such programs often seek to deal on an individual basis with the learner, the better to restrict inputs and interactions. It is obviously poorly suited to work with adolescents who are peer group oriented.

Sex education as the task of parents — this issue is close to the heart of our concern. This belief justifies many agencies in their abdication of responsibility for providing sex education. Many social agencies, as a result of some of the pressures discussed earlier, develop policies which openly reflect the community fears and superstitions about sex. Such fears may cripple the effectiveness of educational programs. The often heard cop-out is that "moral education is the parents job." Such a posture is especially egregious when it occurs on the part of agencies acting as parental substitutes. (SIECUS, 1970)

These common failings command our attention to two dimensions of sex education and training: content and training process. The content must address the entire spectrum of sexual issues. The process must acknowledge that we seek not merely to present information but to aid in the assimilation of that information into an informed code of sexual behavior. The following section offers a framework for implementing these two dimensions in the planning of staff training.

A Framework for Program Planning

Most informed people are aware that sexuality is a pervasive part of human existence. It had varied aspects and manifestations, each of which has significance for our ultimate well functioning as sexual human beings. The SIRIS model proposed by Gochros offers a useful guide in planning sex education programs (1977). SIRIS is an acronym for five significant aspects of sexuality:

*S*ensuality-sex as physical pleasure, whether genital or diffuse
*I*ntimacy-sex as a bonding mechanism between people
*R*eproduction-sex as a procreational activity
*I*dentity-sex as a defining element of self and social roles
*S*exualization - the use of sex to disguise non-sexual motives
   (e.g., rape as sexualized aggression)

These aspects of sexuality need to be considered in any program oriented to adolescent sexual needs. In developing these aspects of sex into a training model, it is useful to conceptualize them into the three traditional educational domains used by social work educators.

Knowledge Domain — the presentation of new ideas or information. Provides for an informed data base about the subject to be considered.

Attitude Domain — exploration of feelings and values on the subject matter presented. Provides for the total integration of the new information into the personal value system of the learner.

Skill Domain — development of new competencies in using the affectively assimilated information. Provides for the application of integrated knowledge to some stated task.

Any of the five SIRIS components can be addressed at any of the training levels. In practice, there is considerable overlap of the three domains, even though they may be conceptualized as distinct. Each may be evaluated differently at the conclusion of training.

It is important to note that different types of training formats differ in their effectiveness in one or another of the domains. Thus, overreliance on a single training mode may result in the types of training errors noted in the SIECUS report.

Developing the Training Program

There are four stages to the development of in-service training programs: needs determination, development of objectives, format selection, and implementation. Evaluation is not identified as a distinct phase of the process, even though it is critical to the success of the training program. As we shall see, the reason for this is that evaluation is embedded in an ongoing process of needs determination.

Needs Determination. Many training programs flounder in this first phase of the process. Accurate needs determination is essential to program success, and its absence almost guarantees failure. It is also the part of the process about which most administrators are most careless.

Let us begin by distinguishing between staff interests, staff needs, and institutional needs.

What usually passes for needs determination in most agencies is someone passing around a questionnaire asking what staff members would like in the way of training. There are several problems with this approach.

1. *We don't know what we don't know.* This is particularly true of sexuality. Those who know the least and are least comfortable with sexuality are the least likely to request training on the subject. It goes without saying that these are precisely the people who most need such training.
2. *The "sending coals to Newcastle" problem.* Once people begin to be aware of an area and are sensitive to it, they may request more and more training on the subject, even past the point of diminishing returns. For example, staff may be good at (and consequently interested in) exploring feelings and emotions. They may thus want more techniques in doing this, even though the institution shows signs of needing increased skills in developing behavioral contracts, setting limits, or some other distinct skill. This is, in a sense, the opposite of the previous issue.
3. *"It must be good, I've heard a lot about it."* Surveys seem to demand a response. Thus, at times staff will insert a request for a type of training about which they had heard positive reports. For example, staff may have heard about "assertion training," and even know of someone who is reputed to be a good "assertion trainer." Therefore, they plop it onto the survey sheet, it fits neatly, and the administrator, the staff member, and everyone else is happy. Please note, however, that at no point has the question come up about whether the staff *needs* assertion training, or even what the expected gains might be. They only know that they have heard of it, and that it "sounds good."

(This is not, by the way, a rap on assertion training. It is an excellent approach, and teaches an important and useful type of behavior. Some of my best friends are assertion trainers.)

If the foregoing are staff interests, how can we recognize staff needs? These are simply noted as performance deficiencies. They represent the failure of staff to accomplish some stated goal or objective. Note that training needs are thus identified in the context of agency objectives, while interests may or may not coincide with objectives. Also note that needs are related to activities that must be performed. Thus, the deficiencies of the staff will most often be noted as skill deficiencies. Knowledge and attitude objectives must be understood as precursors to the development of skills that will enhance staff performance. This is a critical difference between training and education. In education, the learning may take place for its own sake. In training, the learning is always directed toward some ultimate performance expectation.

A final factor to be considered in needs determination is the necessity of taking into account the needs of the total institution rather than the aggregate needs of individual staff members. (This is usually referred to as assuming an administrative perspective, on the apparent belief that only administrators consider the larger picture. This may be because it is usually administrators who are writing about such issues. Here we shall cling to the phrase "institutional perspective," firm in our belief that staff members can and do assume that perspective when they are encouraged to do so.) Issues such as agency accountability, staff or budget pressures, and resource allocation may be addressed in this vein. Often the in-service training tends to focus on the workers at the client interface and ignore other levels of institutional operation. As we shall see, this may well lead to the development of impractical training objectives.

How, then, are we to conduct training needs assessment? The following list of devices offers some ways this task may be undertaken. Note that each is, in the final analysis, addressed to the identification of performance deficiencies. These may be difficult to determine depending largely on how clearly the agency has specified its goals and defined its jobs. A total inability to determine training needs using any or all of these procedures is probably an indication of serious administrative failure to clarify the institutional task. No amount of training is likely to help in this event, since the institution may well not know what it is trying to do.

Surveys and questionnaires. This is the most familiar tool, with the pitfalls discussed above. It is useful, but it is not capable of identifying all types of performance deficiencies. Care must be taken to include all levels of the institution in the survey process. It is often illuminating to poll the residents about what sorts of training they feel the staff needs.

Direct and indirect staff expressions. Staff members frequently gripe about some aspect of their job that is troublesome or time-consuming. Such expressions are good indicators of potential needs, especially when they come from diverse sources.

Observations and interviews. Periodic observation of staff members on the job, or supervisory interviews, may be good sources of data about areas where performance is weak or absent. This is a good way to pick up gaps in staff abilities, which are frequently missed in a survey approach.

Use of records. Institutional records can be a valuable source of information on performance deficiencies. They have the advantage of offering retrospective information, such as occurs when a client experiences a sexual problem, and examination of staff records on the client may reveal how a staff person misperceived or failed to perceive the problem in its emergent phases.

Perusal of records has the added benefit of providing feedback on the total operation of the institution. Too often, clinical records are merely kept for archival purposes. This is unfortunate, since they may serve as valuable data for staff development planning.

Skill inventories. When relatively specific abilities are known to be required for certain necessary tasks, a variety of instruments may be used to determine the presence or absence of the specific skills required, without reference to identified tasks or the necessity of specifying performance deficiencies. For example, if the ability to be confrontive is deemed necessary to aspects of a staff member's job, the scale developed by Carkhuff to measure facilitative confrontation might be employed (Carkhuff, 1969).

Behavioral outcome indicators. Here we refer simply to noting problems (or, more accurately, patterns of problems) that recur. Thus, if clients engage systematically in dysfunctional behaviors, it may be indicative of an identifiable staff deficiency in either planning or some aspects of social interaction facilitation.

To summarize this section briefly, the final responsibility for needs assessment is the administrator's. Needs should be perceived as performance deficiencies, not merely as staff interests. All levels of the institutional system must be considered in needs assessment, and the development of needs priorities must take place in the context of total institutional goal structures.

Development of Objectives. After the training needs have been identified, the next step is to set up the objectives of the training program. Training objectives are similar to educational objectives in general, with the proviso that the training objectives must ultimately address the skill domain discussed earlier. This implies that all knowledge and attitude objectives serve to provide necessary preparation for the development of some needed skill. Knowledge or attitude objectives that do not contribute directly to the development of a job skill should be examined carefully, since they are often included for some purpose that had been poorly thought out. Training time is important, and the inclusion of irrelevant objectives for ancillary or rhetorical purposes will only detract from the effectiveness of the program.

In general, we may say that objectives should be —
1. Precise
2. Measurable
3. Practical
4. Significant

Currently, the literature of education and training is paying much more attention to the first two than the last two. This is a mistaken emphasis, which an in-service trainer should not duplicate.

Precision is what separates objectives from goals. Mager (1962) asks that question of trainers, "How will I know one when I see one?" In others words, what are the *precise* ways in which the staff will be different after training? Precise goals are stated in terms of staff behaviors that will be different as a result of training. For example, an objective might be to increase staff knowledge of birth control so as to counsel with the adolescent residents on this subject. The knowledge base required may be stated with precision, and the ultimate goal of such knowledge giving is to increase the staff time devoted to birth control planning with residents.

Measurability goes hand in hand with precision, since when we state goals with precision it usually involves identifying the measures to be used. Thus, in the example above, we may say that we want all staff to be able to score 100 percent on the sexual knowledge inventory. This would be a knowledge objective measurement. The skill outcome might be measured as an increase of the number of contacts between residents and staff members in which birth control planning is discussed. The ultimate institutional goal then might be served in that the residents undertake informed and responsible birth control planning. The intermediate range of measurability is often the most difficult to frame as a training objective. For example, how does one measure counseling skill? Since the ultimate test of counseling skill is client benefit, and this may take years to reveal itself, we must often settle for approximations. An excellent choice of intermediate measures of counseling effectiveness is available in the work of Truax, et al., who have set up measures of the central traits of effective counselors. By measuring staff performance against the scales developed by Truax and Carkhuff, we are indirectly measuring the effectiveness (or likely effectiveness) of staff counseling. Such measures, when they are validated against the actual demonstrated effectiveness of counselors, may provide useful intermediate measures of staff gains from training.

Significance differs from precision and measurability in that the first two are basic issues. One may have precise and measurable objectives that are either trivial or irrelevant. Precision and measurability are not in themselves guarantees of significance. For example, one might develop precise and measurable goals about sexual anatomy, but the net result would be a training failure of the type described by SIECUS. For training about sexuality to be significant, it must address the multiple aspects of sexuality such as are suggested in the SIRIS model. Further, we must be cognizant of the knowledge, attitude, and skill issues in relation to the subject we discuss. Failure to discuss sexual attitudes will tend to compromise seriously the effectiveness of staff learning. Failure to focus on skill development will result in training that is functionally meaningless, irrespective of any knowledge or attitude gains that might be achieved. Significant objectives must involve both the range of sexual issues and the different levels of learning. Failure to address both dimensions of training will result in suboptimal training programs.

Practicality Can Be a Tricky Issue. It is possible to have objectives that meet the three criteria discussed above, yet still be impractical. For example, a residential facility may have a number of residents who are deeply disturbed about their personal and sexual identities, and there is a clear need for psychotherapy to deal with these concerns. The need may be such that precise and measurable training goals could be established, and certainly the problem is significant. However, the amount of time and resources required to train staff to perform this function may be beyond agency means and, hence, impractical. Even if staff could be trained to do intensive therapy, they might not have time to perform other duties necessary to the operation of the institution. This brings up an important issue in training: *one should never train staff to perform functions to which they will not be assigned.* In addition to being an obvious waste of time and money, it serves to frustrate and alienate the staff who undergo irrelevant training. It also serves to undermine the credibility of the training programs and the administration in general (Herzberg, 1966).

By confining training to specific, attainable objectives, we sometimes find that staff members begin to chafe and become impatient. The narrow range of any given training segment can be offset if staff members are involved in an ongoing needs determination process and long-range planning of staff development programs. By involving staff in their own developmental planning and including them in the overall program we can overcome some of their frustrations. This in turn allows us to focus on the objectives of any given training segment without trying to do too much in a limited time. This long-range planning approach simply reflects good participatory management practices applied to staff development. The payoff is that individual training sessions can retain their focus on well-developed objectives, and the staff can develop a sense of participation and personal development toward a known goal.

The Training Format. The training format should be dictated by the objectives that have been identified. The trainer's credo in this regard is that form follows function. While it may sound obvious to say that the format should be developed to meet the objectives, there are trainers who have techniques (*gimmicks* is probably a better word) that they use irrespective of the setting of objectives. This is an irksome manifestation of Kaplan's Law of the Instrument, which states that if you give a little boy a hammer, everything he sees seems to need hammering. Many sex educators have excellent hammers (multimedia shows, t-groups, beauty pageants, etc.), which are good for some things and not good for others. Just as a hammer makes a poor paintbrush, so does a t-group make a poor vehicle for imparting new information.

Most adult learning is more divergent than convergent. That is, it is usually focused on the expansion and application of information rather than on the input of new information. Adult education calls on the learner to reorganize old concepts, to integrate new ideas into existing schemes, and to explore new linkages created by the learning experience. Knowles refers to this as "adragogical learning," which he contrasts with the older notion of pedagogy (1971). The nature of adragogical learning bears heavily on the design of training programs, as we shall see. Again, this may seem too obvious to mention, until we note the frequency with which sex educators resort to the pedagogical approach of information giving in the form of lectures or electronic substitutes for lectures. (Again, note the SIECUS report on training failures.) Mere presentation of information to a passive audience is not adequate for most training purposes, particularly not in the attitude and skill domains. It has been said that in a lecture room, the only mind working at a reasonable level of efficiency is that of the speaker. Everyone else is operating at a slow idle. To illustrate the point, we may refer to the maxim of a famous consultant named Confucius, who said,

> I *hear* and I forget
> I *see* and I remember
> I *do* and I understand

Knowledge objectives (including what Knowles call "understanding" objectives) are the only materials where the relatively passive techniques are appropriate. Even here, we must use the term *passive* rather carefully. Some of the formats used in imparting information include the following:

Lectures (including televised and film lectures and slides)
Panels, groups, symposia (which are probably overused regarding sexuality)
Readings (which are generally underused in this area)
Observed interviews

These techniques introduce new information to the learner. To promote assimilation of the material into a personal schema, the following techniques may be useful:

Audience participation (questions, discussion, etc.)
Group discussion and interaction
Dramatizations
Group interviews
Problem-solving exercises
Case presentations and analysis
Games and simulations

It is obvious to anyone who ever attended a lecture that the presentation of information does not occur in an emotional vacuum. New ideas or perspectives provoke reactions, and these reactions occur in even the most passive learning situations. However, the trainer should develop learning experiences that promote the assimilation of ideas. As noted in the SIECUS critique, the aim is to open information to multiple interpretations, to encourage pluralistic inputs, and to expand opportunities for application and implication of new ideas. As a general rule, a trainer should *never* offer new information without providing an opportunity to deal with the information.

While the content of training should be dictated by the needs assessment discussed earlier, the following comprehensive checklist of knowledge issues developed by Carrera will provide a reference point for content development (1972).

Anatomy and Physiology
Male and female sex system
Pregnancy and childbirth
Menstruation

Methods of contraception
Biological anomalies
Heredity and sex determination
Sterility-infertility
Human growth and development

Psychosexual and Psychosocial Aspects
Sex differences and sex roles
Sexual concerns of adolescence and other life stages
Sexual socialization processes
Psychosexual development
Role of sex in marriage and family life
Guilt and conflict regarding sexual behavior
Sexual aberrations
Sexual dysfunction
Human sexual response
Sex and drugs
Population growth
Cross-cultural issues
Aging and sexual response
Psychology of family relations: Parent-child relations regarding sex
Sexual abuse

Sexual Behavior and Standards
Dating, courtship, and mate selection
Masturbation
Sexual language (communication)
Petting
Premarital coitus
Nocturnal emissions
Abortion
Homosexuality
Venereal disease
Myths and fallacies
Out of wedlock pregnancy
Western sexual standards: cultural development
Contemporary religious doctrines
Sex dreams and fantasies
Law and sexual behavior
Prostitution

The previous listing is obviously not all-inclusive, but it does point out many areas where the presentation of information will be inextricably linked with the exploration of attitudes. This, in effect, becomes the first phase of the total training process.

Attitudinal Objectives. The process of attitude exploration and clarification begins with the presentation of information. This material is then amplified by using the more experiential techniques listed below. Note that some of these procedures overlap with the information-giving phase discussed above.

Games and simulations (role playing)
Films of explicit sexual activities (coitus, masturbation, oral sex, etc.)
T-groups
Role reversals
Behavioral assignments evoking new perspectives
Personal experience sharing
Case history discussion and analysis
Empathy exercises (identifying feelings in others)
Interaction with guest speakers representing different life-styles

Much of the purpose of affectively oriented training is to expose the trainee to as wide a spectrum of ideas as possible and then to provide an environment where reactions can be safely expressed and explored. The increased awareness of *things* about sex is an aspect of the knowledge domain. The increased awareness of one's *reactions to* those things to which we are exposed is in the attitudinal domain.

Skill Objectives. The training payoff comes in the area of skill improvement in dealing with adolescents and their significant others on the subject of sexuality. Skills in this area might well be organized according to the PLISSIT model developed by Annon and presented in Chapter 9. Annon proposes four levels of intervention with sexual concerns: permission giving, limited information, specific suggestions, and intensive therapy.

Since skill training involves development of active intervention procedures, the training format should be largely experiential. The key techniques include role playing (portraying both client and therapist) behavioral assignments (homework with cases) behavioral drills (empathy exercises, warmth and communication exercises, work on self-disclosure, etc.)

Skill training sessions bring to bear the knowledge, attitude, and skill outcomes from the total training program. In experiential learning, the necessary knowledge base can be reinforced, attitudinal and affective issues can be observed as they emerge in the simulations of casework, and the key traits of warmth and accurate empathy can be developed in work with colleagues, who can offer immediate feedback. The emphasis will be on the general skills of interpersonal helping, since for the most part the techniques used in sexual therapy per se lie outside the scope of most in-service training programs. However, the central traits of nonpossessive warmth, accurate empathy, and genuineness in the interview situation may be developed as the core of effective interpersonal relations between staff and residents on the subject of sexuality. (See Truax and Carkhuff for further discussion of these traits and their clinical implementation.)

Some Final Considerations

In the discussion of in-service training, we have so far avoided the topic that is generally of great concern to those undertaking a training program for the first time: what will I *do* with the people during the training sessions? Most neophyte trainers waste a great deal of concern on the gimmicks of training. A word of reassurance is in order. My own experience in training (and the feedback I receive from colleagues confirms this) is that the techniques of training are of far less importance to the trainees than is the content of the sessions. Relevant information and experiences will go a long way toward satisfying the trainees, and the most sophisticated procedures in the world do not compensate for material that is either irrelevant or impractical. In planning a training session, your time will be much better spent on deciding *what* should be dealt with rather than *how* to deal with it. Ideally, of course, we all want to present the perfect combination of content and process. If we err, however, it is wise to err on the side of content rather than process.

Earlier in this chapter, it was indicated that there were ways in which the apparent disadvantages of formal institutions could be turned to the advantage of staff and residents when dealing with sexuality. One way this can be done is to open up the process of in-service training to include residents as well as staff. By including the residents in the entire process of staff development, soliciting their ideas on the training needs, development of objectives, format selection, and in having them actually participate in the training sessions, a number of things are to be gained.

One gain is that we minimize the role discrepancy between the residents and the staff. By fully involving the residents, we acknowledge that they are the best authorities on what they need and that they have important contributions to make to the operation of the institution. I feel it is better to talk to the residents about what they need than to talk among the staff about what we think they need. Responsible participation by the residents will result in improved training programs, plus carrying the metacommunication that the residents are active participants in the design of their own experience.

A second gain is that the experience of role playing as a vital part of the training process emphasizes the real needs of the residents. By having the residents take the role of helper as well as helpee in role playing, and doing the same with staff, we can improve the empathy that exists between the two. The staff may be able to sense the feeling of the residents, and vice versa.

A third gain is that by conducting the training in an open format, we acknowledge that the staff does not have all the answers, that they too must struggle with difficult issues. It further emphasizes that the residents may have vital information or insights not only about their own sexuality and sexual needs but about sexual concerns of staff members as well.

Finally, the use of an open training format may serve as an important transitional bridge for adolescents who are involved in the transition into adult sexuality. What better way to aid this transition than by treating them as equals in the staff development process? By doing so, perhaps we can overcome the tendency to deal with sexual issues in the secretive and exclusive chambers of adult interactions and to communicate an aura of mistrust by doing so.

I must confess that it takes considerable courage to undertake this approach to training in an open community of staff and residents. In many cases the staff may have serious reservations about undertaking such an effort, thus exposing themselves to observation by their adolescent charges. The inability to do so may simply be one more manifestation of the need of staff for training on sexuality. While a totally open, genuine sharing in the training environment may at first seem an ideal that is unattainable in the real world of role dichotomies and personal insecurities, it may nonetheless be retained as a goal toward which the institution may strive.

BIBLIOGRAPHY

Jack Annon, *The Behavioral Treatment of Sexual Problems: Volume 1, Brief Therapy.* Honolulu, Hawaii: Enabling Systems, 1975.

Bernard Berenson and Robert Carkhuff, *Sources of Gain in Counseling and Therapy.* New York: Holt, Rinehart and Winston, 1967.

Robert Carkhuff and Bernard Berenson, *Beyond Counseling and Therapy.* New York: Holt, Rinehart, and Winston, 1967.

Michael Carrera, "Training the Sex Educator: Guidelines for Teacher Training Institutions," *American Journal of Public Health*, February, 1972.

Catherine Chilman, *Adolescent Sexuality in a Changing American Society.* Washington, D.C.: USDHEW, 1977.

Harvey Gochros, "Human Sexuality," in *Encyclopedia of Social Work*, 17th Issue, Volume I. Washington, D.C.: National Association of Social Workers, 1977.

Irving Goffman, *Asylums.* Garden City, NY: Doubleday, 1961.

Frederick Herzberg, *Work and the Nature of Man.* Cleveland: World Publishing, 1966.

Hisashi Hirayama, "Management of the Sexuality of the Mentally Retarded in Institutions," in D. Kunkel (ed.), *Sexual Issues in Social Work.* University of Hawaii, 1979.

J. R. Kidd, *How Adults Learn.* New York: Association Press, 1973.

Malcolm Knowles, *The Modern Practice of Adult Education: Andragogy vs. Pedagogy.* New York: Association Press, 1971.

Robert Mager, *Preparing Instructional Objectives.* Palo Alto, Fearon, 1962.

Sex Information and Education Council of the United States, *Sexuality and Man.* New York: Charles Scribner's Sons, 1970.

Charles Truax and Robert Carkhuff, *Toward Effective Counseling and Therapy.* Chicago: Aldine, 1967.

Kenneth Wooden, *Weeping in the Playtime of Others.* New York: McGraw-Hill, 1976.

Chapter Eight

SEXUAL CONTACT BETWEEN STAFF AND RESIDENTS

LeRoy G. Schultz

HISTORICALLY, Western society has had a tough time in half-heartedly permitting sexual expression to adults, but society becomes irrational when it tries to control adolescent budding sexual experimentation and sadistic when it combines the control of adolescent sexual expression within its institutions. This triadic mismanagement has resulted in an unwarranted invasion of sexual privacy, a zealous effort to criminalize the young female's sexual development, and community approved interference with normal adolescent sexual integrity. [1,2,3] This sad inheritance forms the foundation for today's ideology on what staff-resident sexual interaction should be.

From today's perspective it may appear that sex-deprivation policy, which has characterized all adolescent institutions, is incompatible with rehabilitation, treatment, and socialization, where, at least in private, professionals decry enforced sexual abstinence and the denial of heterosexual interaction. The adolescent institution was not built out of a fear of an adolescent crime wave but as an idealistic response to moral degeneration fostered by poverty among those ethnic groups who refused the melting pot, by the sordid sexual conditions of the local nonsegregated jails, or simply for those who refused to slide through adolescence gracefully. Adolescent institutions were, in fact, built to treat moral degeneracy (sexual expression) and therefore lusted after sexual reformation as a prime goal. The then current understanding of sexual expression and development makes for grim reading and forms a dark page in social welfare history[4] that should be required reading for all institutional staff. The self-righteousness of zealous sex controllers, always imploring the current best interests of society dogma, was to ban sexual self-stimulation in institutions in 1847 and, in 1893, to open the first institution for disapproved sexually active women, with recommendations for life sentences for sexually active females with poor intelligence.[5,6] The new juvenile court and its social control arms in social welfare institutions reflected and reinforced traditional girl roles, which condoned passivity, helplessness, and incompetence, calling for the restoration of sexual innocence through enforced abstinence. To insure an asexual atmosphere, institutions hired middle-aged staff, married, in good moral standing, capable of the sex-policeman role, and of the same sex as the segregated population. (In 1977 in New York, male guards were removed from female inmate housing, and in 1978 in California, female guards were removed from a boy's institution, by court order.[7])

While the overt sexual sadism of institutions of yesteryear may be gone, remnants of its spirit remain. The Civil Rights Division of the United States Department of Justice in a 1978 survey found that boys were sentenced to solitary confinement for thirty days for sending love notes to a female teacher.[8] Others found that menstruation calanders are posted on female room doors, that residents may not hold hands with anyone, may not comb another person's hair, may not receive a letter from a person of the other sex, may not receive a visit by a person of the other sex, and that females undergo vaginal exams to determine virginity.[9,10] In one large girls' institution visited by the author in 1978, male staff could not interview residents without the roomdoor being 18 inches open, by administrative policy, and new professional staff are requested to call the residents (ages 14-18) girls, not women.

Although institutional reform had progressed to cover due process for patient and resident, prohibiting cruel and unusual punishment, electric behavior modification technique, peonage, and corporal punishment, and while institutions were forced to recognize certain dress and hair styles, neither courts nor institutions have honestly dealt with residents' sexual rights.[11,12,13] This reluctance has had the effect of making every resident's life a sexless one, or one at the whim of administrators' descretion.[14] This sustained judicial, legislative, and administrative recalcitrance towards responsibility for meeting adolescent sexual opportunity in institutions, over time, accounts in large part for the current state of affairs and serves to reinforce the status quo. This takes many forms today, but sexual relations between staff and residents are prohibited everywhere. Institutions tend to resist defining what is permissible short of sexual intercourse or sodomy, seldom informing staff of what they should do sexually.

THE SITUATION TODAY

The author conducted informal interviews with selected staff in various types of adolescent institutions, requesting problems experienced by staff. The seven cases cited here represent the full range of problems that public institutions are encountering and some of their reactions.

Case 1

An institutionalized twelve year old female with an I Q of 65 habitually and manually manipulates the sex organs of male patients and male professionals. The plan to discharge the patient into a community group home is opposed by all staff on the grounds that "she's headed for trouble with boys," with the exception of one male social worker. The male social worker proceeded to work out a promising discharge plan despite peer group opposition and was accused by staff of being sexually obsessed and interested in having sexual relations with the patient. The staff resisted community placement until the services of the institutional ombudsman were invoked by the social worker.

Case 2

In a large state mental hospital, a young male patient habitually makes verbal requests for sexual activity from various female staff. At a staffing of the patient, the majority of professionals recommended censoring the patient and a "couple of days in restraint," to teach him the costs of "sexual harrassment in a nonsexist world." A new female social worker protested this treatment plan, claiming that women in normal life routinely encounter sexually suggestive remarks and body language and that the problem should be handled as it is at large. The staff quickly "cooled out" the new staff member by mentioning that she was over-identifying with the patient, and perhaps her being unmarried was a factor in her sexual interests in the patient.

Case 3

The inmates of a female correctional institution were invited by the superintendent to produce their own choice of a Christmas play attended by inmates and staff. The inmates choose to do their version of *Hair*, which involves a great deal of physical contact between actors and audience. The play was presented, during which there was much hugging, crying, kissing, and stroking, with suggestive body contact of staff and inmates breaking down the wall between the two. Two senior staff were suspended for two days as a disciplinary measure, with references to "lesbianism" and what this looks like to the public.

Case 4

A male graduate student in social work was assigned a seventeen year old female depressed patient as part of his field instruction assignment in a new mental hospital. During treatment for a very recent suicidal gesture, he made voluntary sexual love with the patient, claiming later, in defense, that he was primarily concerned with restoring self-worth in the patient. Hospital administration ejected him from the grounds, claiming he was "sick" and in need of therapy, and besides, a "new hospital hardly needs this."

Case 5

A male recreational therapist formed a close relationship with a teenage boy in an institution for the handicapped. As relief from the boy's overwhelming frustration and depression due to the serious handicap and partial paralysis, the therapist began a sustained pattern of masturbating the boy at the boy's request. Top management engaged in wholesome condemnation and threat of reprisal, while lower level staff give under-the-counter sympathetic approval. (Nurses in some Europeon countries have no problem with masturbating patients. See the 1976 *Report of the National Fund for Research into Crippling Disease*, London.)

Case 6

Ward attendants in a large institution for the mentally retarded take two teenage patients into the bathroom and instruct the two to have intercourse. The awkwardness of the palsied couple incites laughter among bored attendants.

Case 7

A religious institution for troubled girls notes on morning bed check that an attractive, mentally retarded thirteen year old is missing. Later, she was found in another state, pregnant, and stated the institutional gardener had kidnapped her by taking her out through a third floor window on a ladder. The couple lived in various motels until the girl was found. She admitted to sexual involvement with the gardener in the institutional greenhouse.

While no adolescent institution is constitutionally empowered to deny youth sexual opportunity, history indicates a foundation of institutional asexuality and an under-the-counter commitment of staff to assure such asexuality. There is a natural reluctance for administration to volunteer for new responsibilities; many may cite the costs of administering sexual opportunity programs, lack of trained staff, and institutions intentionally built without privacy. The state has consistently limited its role to protector from sexuality, being sensitive to many years of feedback indicating that youth do not want just protection, but participation.

Minors are strongly influenced by our liberated sexual culture in which sexual expression is glamorized, worthy of pursuing, a sign of maturity, and depicted as adult fun. Increases in health and nutrition have resulted in earlier menstruation for girls. Minors have been exposed by the media (almost all adolescent institutions have television now) to prostitution, lesbianism, divorce, different sexual life-styles, sexual humor, abortion, and soap operas saturated with romantic sexuality — all of which combine to produce a different and new sexual atmosphere more sophisticated than in the past. What adolescents do not know about sexual expression is provided by powerful, all-pervasive peer group discussion.

Several recent, reliable studies of the sexual behavior of minors reveal the following:

1. At age 15 years, 18% of American white girls have had sexual relations; female blacks were 38% sexually active by age 15 years.[15]
2. At age 7 many black girls have had or witnessed sexual relations if they live in ghettos.[16]
3. By age 12 years or younger, 13% of all females have had sexual relations and by age 15 it rises to 56%.[17]
4. The average age of first intercourse was 12.8 years, with 15% of boys reporting sexual intercourse with girls under age 9.[18]

To think that adolescents leave their sexual pasts at the gate as they enter the institution is maliciously naive, as is the urge to deprive suddenly those who have been sexually active. Minors learn of the sexual pluralism of today, the thirst for variety and experimentation, and that no person's sexual value system is necessarily better than someone elses.

Aside from the normal sexual patterns that minors bring with them, there are benefits of a therapeutic nature in some types of sexual touching,[19, 20, 21] in close staff-resident relationships,[22] and and possibly some physical health benefits for males in retarding certain diseases through sexual activity.[23, 24] Because one's self-concept is so closely interwoven with sexual identity, forces that threaten sexual identity also threaten personal identity. The denial of sexuality can have a destructive effect not only upon one's sex life but also on one's image and interpersonal relationships.

Recent court decisions in a number of states have forced institutions to acknowledge the social-sexual needs of residents and to provide some opportunities for getting together. Courts have ordered institutions for the retarded in New York and Alabama and juvenile institutions in Texas to provide opportunities for residents to meet and mingle with the other sex and to provide *regular* contact in a variety of settings.[25]

In addition, there has been a change in philosophy resulting in a liberalization of so-called statutory rape laws in the various states. Five states now allow girls age fourteen or older to have sexual intercourse, in effect, with boys under age eighteen, and some states, in effect, allow girls over age sixteen to have intercourse with males under age twenty-one, while many states set the absolute age of sexual consent at sixteen: at least such male's partners cannot be charged with statutory rape.[26] However, three states may hold staff on statutory rape charges following voluntary sexual intercourse if a consenting resident is under age sixteen years (New Mexico and New Hampshire) or under age fifteen (South Carolina).[26]

Adolescent residents in institutions, unless reasonably contraindicated, should be permitted maximum sexual choice with consenting peers through joint policy-making arrangements in institutional governance. Institutions should not add insult to injury in further sexual shaming of adolescent residents, in stigmatizing with the moralistic dogma labeled "sexually acting-out," or in pressuring through restrictive cues supporting yesterday's taboo.

SEXUALITY AND INSTITUTIONAL STAFF

Although it sounds obvious, it bears repeating: staff are sexual beings also. They bring to their jobs and professional roles personal sexual values and comfort levels, or they may have only their rememberances of their own adolescence to guide them in staff-resident relations. While institutions vary in creating a sexual or an asexual climate, in general, close living, relating, and sharing have a powerful sexual impact on staff as well. The institution by its vary nature creates a heightened need for sexual expression through boredom, the sexual peak of residents' lives, and the lack of sensitivity and normal touching behaviors. There is little to validate a resident as a sexually worthy person, and some well-meaning staff may choose to intervene.

Many staff may come from social, ethnic, or racial backgrounds different from those of the residents, causing strain, misunderstanding, and confusion. Residents may be aware of staff dating each other, visiting each other at night if housed on the institutional grounds, inciting rumor and gossip, all adding to a charged sexual atmosphere. Very few staff feel comfortable in using their own experiences as resident education or as role modeling. However, many new staff or volunteers may differ in age only by a few years from residents and may have more in common with residents than with older staff. The new, young professional may sense that the individual life cycle is being freed from the tight sexual timetable of the past, that the age of puberty has dropped, that adolescents attain intellectual and physical maturity at an earlier age, perhaps causing young staff to identify more with residents than staff. Older staff and administrators may have suspicions of a conspiracy or collaboration between young staff and residents against older staff. Such division of staff can be exploited by some residents. Some residents are more sexually sophisticated than staff, thus causing staff self-consciousness and resentment with feelings of inadequacy. Staff may simply not know how to respond to seductive behaviors by residents.[27]

New, younger staff members may naively attempt to change the asexual environment of the institution by themselves on a case-by-case basis, again forming a collusive relationship with selected residents. This usually leaks out to all, with subsequent feelings of hostility and stigmentizing of those who break ranks, and the fragile hold that staff have built up over the years is shattered. Residents and staff may gossip about one another in a viscious scheme, with administration playing both ends against the middle. Older staff and administration may then personalize the professional's concern for resident sexual welfare and turn it back on the professional before peers, as seen in several of the cited cases. Staff attitudes can limit sexual expression. Staff are as susceptible as anyone to adolescent and sexual sterotypes, prejudices, and anxiety, but unlike the general public they have a job to do that is becoming increasingly inconsistent with this negative view, causing additional strain. Adding to the burden are large staff case loads that may force legitimate concern for sexual welfare aside or make it secondary.

STAFF-RESIDENT SEXUAL RELATIONS

Seductive behavior, under a shifting definition of acceptance, is a socially desirable skill that our socioerotic space reinforces. One is not considered mature unless he or she has developed a suitable seduction repertoire and adequate defense to counter unwanted seduction. Seductive behavior is a form of adolescent flirtation, which ultimately form pathways to mature sexual relating, enhancing intimacy and affection, clearing signals and body language, and supporting self-esteem. Thus, seduction management becomes a learned, crucial interpersonal tool. Sociosexual scripting of male and female involves learning the give and take of seductive encounters in a sexually bountiful world, albeit each sex somewhat differently, and both staff and older residents carry such sexual scripting into institutional relationships. Thus both resident and staff are subject to sexual temptation. What one does with seductive feelings and their actions differentiates a professional relationship from other types. New, young staff, products of a different sexual revolution, may find yesterday's definition of erotic transference and countertransference and past management prescriptions as unnecessarily harsh, restrictive, and plain inhuman. Admonishments to abide by a professional code of ethics or some ancient sex code or to refrain from all erotic contact do little to guide staff or residents, do little to reduce ambiguity-induced anxiety, and do not fit the new humanistic values. The view that children and adolescent girls have both sexual needs and the right to fulfill them strikes many as more trouble than it's worth. It is the younger staff to whom residents may take their sexual and affectionate needs, rather than the older "watch out for boys" mother figures. In addition, some new treatment techniques involve touching and higher levels of intimacy with clients, with few guidelines for staff.[28] While staff may possess many treatment skills, they do not know what to do when the resident sexualizes them, short of wholesale condemnation of the "seducer."

At present, there is no legal justification for resident/staff sexual intercourse either as sex therapy or sex education, and there is much societal condemnation. No matter how justified such methods are in theory or in terms of efficacy, staff are doomed to corrective action, such as termination of employment and possible jail sentence under a wide variety of protective but ancient laws: contributing to the delinquency of a minor, corruption of the morals of youth, fornication, lewd behavior, and a vague batch of legal nay-sayings. No matter what the circumstances, the word *exploitation* will be invoked. Society has so narrowly defined sexual activity that its use for any other reason will not be tolerated. Much the same holds for the use of surrogates or clinical prostitutes in treatment, no matter how effective these are for adults.[29] In short, since institutions were built on a foundation of punishment, including a nonsexual life-style for residents, for staff to actually engage in sexual relations invites considerable censure. Adolescent residents in public institutions cannot sign treatment contracts, and under *pariens patria* the state is their parent, so natural parents cannot sign for them even if consenting to treatment involving erotic contact. Adolescents in institutions must seek sexual satisfaction only from peers, even though such behavior is now prohibited in most institutions.

SUGGESTED CHANGES

1. Since privacy is essential for comfortable sexual activity, most of the older, larger institutions, particularly custodial and

correctional, must be abandoned, or architectual redesign will be required. All new, and hopefully smaller, institutions constructed in the future should take personal privacy directly into the brick and morter, with soundproof walls and human social space, compatable with safety and institutional function.
2. Staff and administration should abandon phrases such as "sexual acting-out," "nymphomania," and "premature whores." These phrases are simply reflections of staff personal values, or diagnostic masking for social control, and should be stricken from the professional vocabulary. A realistic evaluation of sexual patterns of adolescents is sorely needed, with sexual rights held uppermost. Indeed, an Insitutional Bill of Rights is required, based on an honest awareness of adolescent sexual patterns with consideration given to social class and minority differences and preferences.
3. Staff may require institutes and in-house workshops in which information on sexual needs and practices is provided, coupled with attitudinal restructuring, sexual desensitization, anxiety-reduction techniques, and the skills required for healthy reaction to resident's seductive strategies. Staff unable to respond to required changes should be reassigned to less destructive roles. Job descriptions within civil service systems must directly acknowledge worker responsibility for sexual welfare, both protectively and in terms of participation.
4. Staff apprehended in sexual relations with residents for the first time should not automatically be terminated. The employer should first provide psychotherapy for such staff with emphasis on seduction management, positive use of resident sexual need, and self-control. If direct use of sexual self has therapeutic value in the judgement of certain staff, this position and its defense should be discussed at staff meetings before usage so that its total impact can be acknowledged and addressed by all, and transference-counter transference can be controlled.

While a New Mexico court (1978) upheld, in effect, the right of a fourteen year old boy to acquire a sex education through sexual intercourse with an older women, and while a New York family court judge (1978) upheld the right of a fourteen year old girl to prostitute herself, and while nurses may masturbate sexually deprived patients in some countries, it may be some time before professionals gain the required skills to use these methods effectively. It appears very few professional or layity are ready to accept staff-resident sexual intercourse as therapeutically defensible. This is no excuse from resexualizing the social space of institutions up to that limit, however.

5. Preventing staff-resident sexual intercouse or other direct sexual contact should be the responsibility of staff supervisors, who also need the skill, knowledge, and values regarding normal adolescent sexual development and needs. This should include the maintenance of a reasonable institutional moral code and an awareness of what impedes open staff communication on sexual matters. If staff are to move beyond a defensive stance to reasonable involvement, they in turn must have some kind of emotional support built into the institutional system to help them deal with healthy coping.

6. Court decisions from outside the institutional organization are forcing sociosexual changes on institutions. Implementing court decisions is another matter. The complexity of large organizations is as important a factor in non compliance as is willful resistance. Controlling internal and external units responsible for implementation may be too much for any administrator in terms of cooperation and coordination. As a result, a realistic appraisal of the feasibility of any institutional reform proposal must include the following:
    a. Identifying various organizations, departments, staff member and private groups whose cooperation on compliance is required.
    b. Ascertainment of the needs and interests of those groups to determine whether and to what degree the proposed policy will threaten those need and interests.
    c. Evaluation of the capacity and standard operations procedure of the various relevent groups for their adaptibility to the recommended change.[30]

These constraints on court-induced institutional change in sexual matters indicate the need for the institution itself to take more of a leadership role, hopefully, with support of the institutional ombudsman. Perhaps creating a new offense, "Institutions in Need of Supervision," will not just have a coercive impact for change but will lend the courts power to help institutions demand resources necessary for implementation from their budgetary authority.

7. Perhaps the most powerfully favorable impact on adolescent sexual freedom will result from the continued deinstitutionalization movement, the removing of so-called status offenses from juvenile court jurisdiction, enforcement of "least restrictive environment" policy and the "best sexual interests of the child" ideology, rather than sexual fulfillment resulting from resident-staff sexual interaction. Needed is a sexual affirmitive action policy, as there is no justifiable state interest served by sexually neutered adolescent institutions.

The deprivation policy of public institutions is unjustly severe and destructive. There is a disheartening lack of discussion of the issue. This silence gives the facade of principled adolescent welfare policy. If the human costs of our desexualization policy and implementation towards institutionalized youth are taken into account (loss of dignity, loss of freedom of choice, invasion of privacy, loss of individuality), they are tantamount to criminal schemes against the developing adolescent. Now, when we speak of the quality of life, social indicators, health indicators, or therapeutic community, the indices will take into account healthful sexual expression of all.

REFERENCES

1. D. Rothman, *Discovery of the Asylum*. Boston: Little, 1971.
2. A. Platt, *The Child Savers: The Invention of Delinquency*. Chicago: U of Chicago Pr, 1969.
3. S. Schlossman, S. Wallach, The crime of precocious sexuality: Female delinquency in the progressive era. *Harvard Educational Review, 48(1):* 65-94, 1978.
4. L. Schultz, The sexual abuse of children and minors: A short history of legal control efforts. In L. Schultz (Ed.), *The Sexual Victimology of Youth*. Springfield: Thomas, 1980.
5. P. Mennel, *Thorns and Thistles: Juvenile Delinquency in the U.S., 1825-1940*. Hanover, NH: U of New England Pr, 1973, pp. 71, 99.

6. W. Lewis, *From Newgate to Dannemora*. New York: Macmillan, 1965, p. 131.
7. R. Smith, Sexual privacy. *Juris Doctor*, January 1978, pp. 19-23.
8. DHEW-OHDS, *Child Abuse and Neglect in Institutions* (78-30160). Washington, U.S. Govt. Print. Office, 1978, p.2.
9. K. Rodgers, For her own good. *Law and Society Review*, 6:223-246, 1972.
10. K. Wooden, *Weeping in the Playtime of Others*. New York: McGraw, 1976.
11. S. Krantz, *The Law of Corrections and Prisoner Rights*. St. Paul: West Pub, 1976.
12. A. Stone, *Mental Health and Law* (DHEW -ADM 76-16). U.S. Govt. Print. Office, 1975.
13. R. Burt, The therapeutic use and abuse of state power over adolescents. *Current Issues in Adolescent Psychiatry*, 1973, pp.243-251.
14. J. Jacobs, E. Steele, Sexual deprivation and penal policy. *Cornell Law Review, 62(2)*:289-312, 1977.
15. M. Zelnick, J. Kanter, Sexual and contraceptive experience of young unmarried women in U.S. 1976 and 1971. *Family Planning Perspective, 9(2)*: 55-73, 1977.
16. J. Ladner, B. Hammond, *Socialization into Sexual Behavior*. New York: Society for the Study of Social Problems, 1967.
17. R. Sorenson, *Adolescent Sexuality in Contemporary America*. New York: World, 1973, p.214.
18. M. Finkel, D. Finkel, Sexual and contraceptive knowledge, attitudes and behavior of male adolescents. *Family Planning Perspectives, 7(6)*: 356-359, 1975.
19. D. Krieger, Therapeutic touch: The imprimatur of nursing. *American Journal of Nursing, 75:*784-787, 1975.
20. L. Davis, Touch, sexuality and power in residential settings. *British Journal of Social Work, 5(4)*:398-411, 1976.
21. M. Hollender, The need or wish to be held, *Archives of General Psychiatry*, 22:445-453, May 1970.
22. R. Morris, Female delinquency and relational problems. *Social Forces*, October 1964, pp.117-121.
23. J. Brecher, Sex, stress and health. *International Journal of Health Services, 7(1)*:89-101, 1977.
24. K. Money, Physical damage caused by sexual deprivation in girls. *Medical Hypothesis, 4:*141-148, 1978.
25. A. Neir, Sex and confinement. *Civil Liberties Review, 5(1)*:6-16, 1978.
26. L. Schultz, The age of sexual consent: Fault, friction and freedom. In L. Schultz (Ed.), *Sexual Victimology of Youth*. Springfield: Thomas, 1980.
27. L. Schultz, J. McGrath, Teaching seduction management skills. In L. Nelson, E. Anderson, *Helping People*. Johnson City: East Tennessee State University Press, 1979, pp.267-270.
28. L. Schultz, A survey of social workers' attitudes and use of body and sex psychotherapies. *Clinical Social Work Journal, 3:*90-99, 1975.

29. M. Gorelick, A simple course in sex. *Human Behavior, 2:*56-57, 1973.
30. B. Ruback, The sexually intergrated prison: A legal and policy evaluation. *American Journal of Criminal Law, 3(3):*301-339,

PART III
CLINICAL APPROACHES

Chapter Nine

A PRACTICAL APPROACH TO DAY TO DAY SEXUAL PROBLEMS

Jack S. Annon and Craig H. Robinson

THERE are a growing number of psychologists, social workers, psychiatrists, physicians in various specialties, ministers, marriage counselors, and others whose training and experience qualify them to deal with sexual problems. However, there are also a number of ways in which institutional staff may be of immediate assistance to adolescents with sexual concerns. This chapter will outline some of them. Initially, the chapter will offer some general suggestions for preparation for dealing with sexual matters, along with some specific counseling tips for dealing with adolescents. A model will then be described for providing direct assistance to adolescents with sexual concerns.

PREPARATION

Background in the Sexual Area

The more information that you have regarding human sexual behavior the more confidence that you may have in offering assistance. In addition to what you have learned from the preceding chapters, the following suggestions might be helpful.

Readings. Self-study can be extremely useful in acquiring basic knowledge in this area, and a number of informative books will be discussed later in this chapter. Sharing the information you obtain with your colleagues will also aid in the retention and application of such knowledge. For example, you could start your own sex book of the week, or month, club with interested staff members, where you read an article or book in your area of interest and then report your findings to others in the group for discussion and comparison with what they have read.

Lectures, Courses, and Seminars. Many colleges and universities offer specific courses in various aspects of sexuality, which may be available to you. In addition, your particular institution might consider inviting appropriate speakers from these academic settings or other community agencies to address your staff.

Films. Viewing sexually explicit films designed for educational purposes is often an excellent way of gaining information about the broad range of human sexual behaviors that exists across cultures as well as within a culture. Such films may also increase your awareness of sex practices divergent from your own and, hopefully, increase your tolerance and acceptance of sexual behaviors and values different from yours.

Counseling Tips

The Setting. It is not too important *where* you talk with the adolescent as long as there is some measure of privacy. Talking with adolescents in an office, hallway, or dining room crowded with their peers will certainly not promote much dialogue. On the other hand, talking with them in a deserted hallway or quietly in the corner of the dining room where you will not be heard by others may be private enough for a helpful discussion.

The Initial Approach. Once you are in a discussion with an adolescent, it is important to select an opening with which you feel comfortable. For example, with a teenage male who casually mentions that a lot of his friends seem to be "sexually hung up," you might say "Well, it certainly is common for many young men to have a lot of questions about sex. Do you have any questions or problems in this area that you would like to ask about? I'm certainly not an expert, but if I don't know the answers I do know where I can find them." The main point here is that it is not so important *what* you say as *how* you say it. If you appear nervous by avoiding his eyes, fidgeting, or looking over your shoulder, you probably won't instill much confidence. Time is another factor in such a situation.

If the teenager does respond with a question and you look at your watch and say that you really don't have time to discuss it then, but perhaps later in the week, you will certainly reduce the chances of his approaching you again. If you do not have sufficient time to follow through, do not open up the area for discussion. If you should be caught at an inconvenient moment, then let him know that you would like to discuss it more fully with him, and set a definite appointment at the first available time. It is also important *not* to continue to probe or press him if he responds that he does *not* have a problem or question, even though it appears obvious to you that he does. He is the best judge of when he is ready to talk about such matters. The important point is not to press but to be sure to let him know that *if* he should ever have any questions in the future, you are available to talk with him. This will allow him time to think about the matter, and he will probably contact you again in the near future. On the other hand, suppose he does respond that he has a problem. What do you do? You might remember the three *L* s of counseling: listening, language, and labeling.

Listening. One of the most common errors — even among professionals — is failure to really listen to what the adolescent has to say without interrupting or jumping to conclusions. Such failure to listen increases the chances of offering inappropriate suggestions based on unfounded assumptions. Often, an adolescent may not have a specific problem but just wants the opportunity to check something out with someone who might know more about the matter. Further, do not assume that what the adolescent says is actually the problem. He or she may be telling you about someone else's problem, or even testing you to see how you respond to a minor matter before bringing up the major concern. Typical follow-up questions might be; Does that bother you? How do you feel about it? It that a problem for you or your friend? It is also helpful to avoid questions that can be answered by a simple yes or no. You might ask a hundred questions this way and obtain very little information. You might use the counselor's most favorite prompt: "Please, tell me more about that."

Language. What language should you use when talking about sexual matters with an adolescent? Should you use medical or technical terms, or should you use the teenage slang of the day? There are dangers with both approaches. In the first case, the teenagers may not understand what you are talking about; rather than ask, they may just pretend that there is no problem after all. In the second approach, many adolescents may feel that you are putting them on and being condescending or ridiculing them. In general, it is usually wise to initially use the language that *you* feel comfortable with and then negotiate. If you use terms such as *coitus* or *sexual intercourse* and the adolescent talks about *balling* or *screwing*, you might finally both agree on using *loving*. However, be certain that you both have the same definitions. To avoid misunderstandings, it is important to ask for *descriptions* of behavior rather than labels where you might assume one meaning and the adolescent another.

Labeling. Labeling adolescents or their behavior is not helpful for understanding and helping them with their problems. This is true for a number of reasons. Labeling adolescents as delinquent does not tell anything specific about their behavior, thoughts, or feelings in relation to their specific problems. Labeling adolescents may make assumptions about them that may not actually apply. Labeling usually implies that the adolescent behaves that way under all conditions at all times. It is now well established that, other variables being equal, an adolescent's behavior in a particular situation is largely determined by past experiences in similar situations. Without further clarification by *description*, labels such as delinquent, queer, macho, hyperactive, or passive are not helpful and do not suggest what to actually do about a specific problem.

To be helpful to adolescents, you might not only give up using such labels yourself, but you may also attempt to help them do likewise. Helping them to use descriptions and give up labeling can be a very powerful therapeutic experience in itself. This is true because in a given culture, many labels automatically bring out a negative emotional response on the part of the persons to whom they are applied, whether self-applied or given by others. For example, there are distinct therapeutic advantages in helping an adolescent girl learn to say "I have not had a chance to learn how to experience an orgasm yet" as opposed to "I am frigid," or "I've had a sexual experience with someone of the same sex" as opposed to I'm a homosexual" (assuming he or she is presenting this as a problem); conversely, "I've had a sexual experience with someone of the opposite sex" as opposed to "I'm macho," or "I'm having a problem in getting an erection" as opposed to "I'm impotent."

There is wide disagreement by professionals on various definitions in the sexual area. For example, different authorities have variously defined *impotence* as failure of erection, failure of orgasm, inability to perform the sexual act, a need for perverse fantasies, the inability to conclude successfully the act of intercourse to the satisfaction of the male, imagining that he is with someone other than his partner — to name only a few. What does an adolescent mean when he says he is a quick trigger or that he is suffering from premature ejaculation? Some authorities call this a form of impotence, while others do not. It has also been described as ejaculation before vaginal entry, before erection, during vaginal entry, after vaginal entry, prior to the completion of four strokes, anytime before the male is ready, or even anytime before the female is ready.

What does an adolescent girl mean when she calls herself an ice box or says that she is frigid? Definitions by various experts are impotence in the female, being abnormally adverse to sexual intercourse, lack of vaginal orgasm, lack of any orgasm, lack of arousal, or complete lack of a pleasurable response to erotic stimuli of any kind. This label has been further compounded by the addition of a multitude of qualifying terms such as true, pseudo, primary, secondary, relative, temporal, and situational. When the so-called experts do not agree on what they mean by these labels, is it any wonder that nonprofessional people have similar difficulties? Hopefully, the point is clear: labeling adolescents or their behavior is not helpful in understanding or offering them assistance. It is also hoped that the remedy is equally clear: ask the adolescent to *describe* the problem behavior as clearly as possible instead of labeling it.

Value Labels. Another closely related area is the use of such value labels by adolescents as good or bad, and right or wrong. Adolescents use these value judgements to describe their own behavior; by doing so, they often compound the anxiety and conflict associated with their problem. Quite often they may ask someone in a position of authority if their behavior is bad or good, right or wrong, normal or abnormal. If you want to be of assistance you will avoid the use of these value labels and help them do the same. You can avoid the use of these terms based on an absolute external system by using descriptive terms in relation to their stated goals. In other words, *instead of labeling a specific behavior as bad, good, right or wrong, you can look at the behavior in terms of their goals and ask, Is that particular behavior going to be useful or not useful, or helpful or not helpful in reaching their goals?*

In using such terms as *useful* or not, *helpful* or not, *appropriate* or not in direct reference to the adolescent's goals, you avoid the hazards and difficulties associated with external value systems. Even more important, you may provide a model for adolescents, who now may have a more productive method for evaluating their own behavior. This does not mean that you must give up your personal value system. There may be times when the adolescent's goals may come into direct conflict with your value system, and it is then your responsibility to clearly inform them of this and to refer them elsewhere if appropriate.

Assume that you have prepared yourself for counseling through the use of readings, lectures, seminars, and films. Assume, too, that you are talking with an adolescent in privacy, you are maintaining eye contact without fidgeting, with sufficient time, and that you have used a comfortable opening and have learned how to listen, negotiated on language, and have avoided labeling. The adolescent has carefully described his or her sexual concern and waits expectantly. What do you do? What you may do will be described in the next section by presentation of a model for offering possible assistance. How well you do will depend upon your preparation.

AN ASSISTANCE MODEL

There are numerous systems of therapy upon which specialists may base their treatment procedures for helping people with sexual problems; however, there are relatively few models available to other helping professionals from different backgrounds, training, and experiences that can aid them in providing assistance to others in the sexual area. Such a model ought to be comprehensive and flexible so that it can be adapted to whatever time is available as well as be used by people with diverse training. The model also ought to allow for a range of assistance choices geared to the level of competence of the particular staff person. It would also be helpful if the model offered a framework for screening out and treating those problems which may be responsive to brief approaches and those which may require more intensive treatment.

After devising and testing a number of approaches in different settings with a variety of people with diverse problems, a model that looked promising was finally developed and shared, taught to others, and refined; then, a final, workable scheme seemed to emerge. Since then this model has been offered to others in the helping professions via lectures, workshops, and training programs, as well as through audiotape cassettes (Annon & Robinson, 1977; Hindle, 1978), articles (Annon, 1976b; Pion & Annon, 1975), and books (Annon, 1975, 1976a). It appears that a number of people in the helping professions with diverse training have found it to be useful, as it is currently being offered to and used by psychologists (Annon, 1975, 1976a); physicians (Annon & Robinson, in press a; Croft, 1976); such specialists as obstetricians, gynecologists, and urologists (Hindle, 1978; Pion & Annon, 1975); social workers (Gochros, 1978; King, 1977); rehabilitation specialists (Annon & Robinson, in press a); sex therapists (Annon & Robinson, 1978; Fischer & Gochros, 1977); family life and human sexuality teachers (Daniel, 1979); and college students with a variety of majors (Annon & Robinson, in press b and c; Kelly 1979). In addition to the model being used to assist individuals and couples with a wide range of sexual concerns, it has also been applied to women's groups (Morton & Pion, 1976) as well as to heterosexual couples' groups with various sexual dissatisfactions (Baker & Nagata, 1978). It is hoped that this model will find equal applicability for staff working with the sexual concerns of institutionalized adolescents.

THE PLISSIT MODEL

As an aid to memory, this approach is referred to as the PLISSIT model or, more accurately, P-LI-SS-IT. The model provides for four levels of help, and each letter or pair of letters designates a suggested method for handling particular sexual concerns. The four levels are *P*ermission − *L*imited *I*nformation − *S*pecific

A Practical Approach to Sexual Problems 111

*S*uggestions — *I*ntensive *T*herapy. A visual presentation of the proposed model may help clarify how it may be applied in a variety of settings. Let each line in Figure 9-1 represent the different presenting sexual concerns that a staff person encounters over time. Depending upon profession, setting, and specialty, these problems may represent what one meets in one day, one month, one year, or even one lifetime.

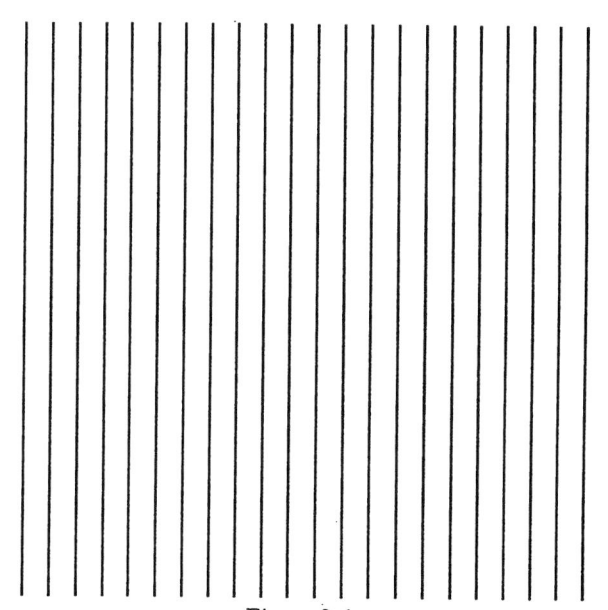

Figure 9-1

Figure 9-2 depicts the theoretical application of the P-LI-SS-IT model to these sexual concerns. As Figure 9-2 further illustrates, the first three levels can be viewed as *brief therapy* as contrasted with the fourth level, *intensive therapy*.

Brief Therapy
- P
- LI
- SS

Intensive Therapy
- IT

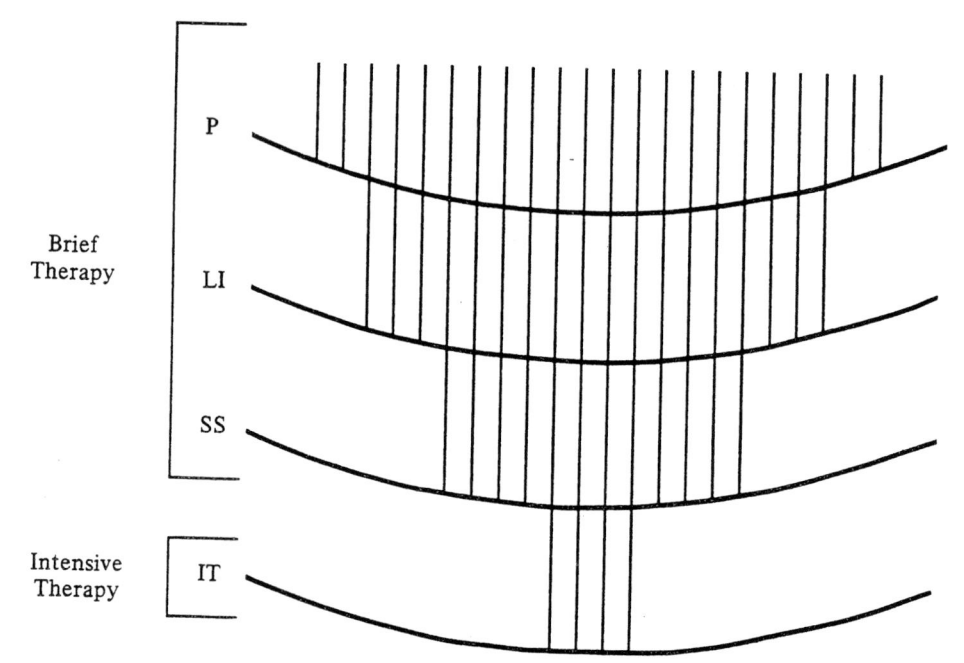

Figure 9-2

The use of this model has a number of distinct advantages. It may be used in a variety of settings and adapted to whatever time is available. Theoretically, each descending level of approach requires increasing degrees of knowledge, training, and skill on the part of the person using it. The model thus allows individuals to gear this approach to their own particular level of competence. This also means that people now have a plan that aids them in determining when referral elsewhere is appropriate. Most important, the model provides a framework for discriminating between those problems which require intensive therapy and those which may be responsive to brief therapy.

How many levels of approach you will feel competent to use will directly depend upon the amount of interest and time you are willing to devote to expanding your knowledge, professional training, and skill at each level. The remainder of this section will be devoted to brief, practical suggestions on how to apply these levels of assistance.

PERMISSION

Sometimes, all that adolescents may want to know is that they are normal, that they are okay, that they are not perverted, deviated, or abnormal, and that there is nothing wrong with them. Many times people are not bothered by the specific behavior in which they are engaging, but they *are* bothered by the thought that there may be something wrong or bad with what they are doing. Frequently, they just want someone to act as a sounding board for checking out their concerns. In other cases, they may need to know that they are not alone or unusual in their concerns and that many people share them. Reassurance that they are normal and permission to continue doing exactly what they have been doing is sufficient in some cases to resolve what might become a very major problem. Thus, permission giving can be seen as a preventative measure as well as a treatment technique. Permission giving will certainly not resolve all sexual problems, or even most such problems, but it may resolve some, as Figure 9-2 suggests. Furthermore, it has the advantage of being useful in almost any setting at any time, while taking minimal preparation on your part. Finally, it may be used to cover a number of areas of concern, e.g. covert behaviors such as thoughts, fantasies, dreams, and feelings as well as overt behaviors.

It is not at all unusual for adolescents to express a variety of worries regarding certain sexual dreams, thoughts, or fantasies they may have had. To be told that many others have the same or similar experiences can be highly reassuring and therapeutic. For example, adolescents (as well as adults) often have occasional dreams involving sexual activity with a wide variety of people such as friends, relatives, parents, brothers, and sisters. At times, the dreams may also involve sexual activity with the same sex, even though the dreamer may never have had (or wanted) such actual experiences. Reassurance that such dreams are entirely within the normal range and are not unusual or indicative of abnormality, is usually sufficient to relieve the anxiety or guilt associated with them. Often such permission giving is also sufficient to stop the recurring sexual dream that was associated with anxiety, just as it can alleviate the persistent thought or fantasy.

A great number of young people are frequently very anxious and/or guilty over their masturbatory patterns and may be greatly relieved to be given permission to engage in such activity. Other areas of concern where permission giving might be helpful are too numerous to delineate here, though by now they are probably self-evident.

It must be emphasized, however, that with permission giving (as well as any other therapeutic strategy) it is the responsibility of the staff person to make sure the adolescent is fully informed about the sexual activity in question, especially regarding any potential negative personal and societal consequences.

If permission giving is not sufficient to resolve the adolescent's concern and if you do not have sufficient time or relevant knowledge and/or skills, then this is the time to refer the adolescent elsewhere. On the other hand, if you do have appropriate time, knowledge, and skills, then you may combine your permission giving with the second level of assistance.

LIMITED INFORMATION

In contrast to permission giving, which is basically telling adolescents that it is all right to continue doing what they have been doing or *not do* what they do not wish to do, limited information is seen as providing them with specific factual information directly relevant to their particular sexual concern. It may result in their continuing to do what they have been doing, or it may result in their doing something different. For example, one of the authors encountered a young man whose major concern was a feeling of inadequacy because he considered his penis too small in comparison with other males. He had withdrawn from any social contact, was depressed over his situation, and was contemplating trying to obtain surgery to correct his "deficient" penis. He was provided with the usual information that can be given in such cases, e.g. the foreshortening effect of viewing his own penis as compared to looking across at other males; the lack of correlation between flaccid and erect penis size except for tendency for the smaller flaccid penis to become longer in the erect state than the longer flaccid penis; the average length of the female vagina as being 3 to 4 inches; the few nerve ending deep inside the vagina, etc. A few minutes of such relevant information giving was sufficient to change his outlook, and within two months he was socially popular and involved in a close sexual relationship with a young woman to whom he eventually became engaged. Of course, it is impossible to predict what might have happened had he not been given such relevant information, but it seems likely that his situation might have progressively deteriorated. Thus, as with permission giving, providing limited information may also be seen as a preventative measure as well as a treatment technique. Also, in the situation described, the client was given permission to have his concern and to accept his own body, but he was not directly given permission to avoid or seek out sexual contact with women. By supplying relevant information, he was provided with an opportunity to change his behavior if he chose to do so.

It should be pointed out that limited information is usually given in conjunction with permission giving. While each may be used as separate levels, there may obviously be considerable overlap between the two. Furthermore, both can be used in conjunction with the remaining two levels of assistance. However, because each descending level of treatment usually requires more time, knowledge, experience, and skill for most effective application, each level is presented and discussed separately.

Other areas in which limited information giving can be particularly helpful to the sexually troubled adolescent may include masturbation, unwanted pregnancies, common homosexual and heterosexual activities, sexually transmitted disease, and menstruation. As with the previous level of treatment, if limited information is not sufficient to resolve the adolescent's concern, and if you do not have sufficient time or relevant knowledge and/or skills, then this is the time to refer the adolescent elsewhere.

SPECIFIC SUGGESTIONS

In contrast to permission and limited information giving, which generally do not require people to take any active steps to change their behavior unless they choose to, specific suggestions are direct attempts to help them to change their behavior to reach their stated goals. This is done from within a brief therapy framework, which means that the approach is time and problem limited.

As with the previous levels of assistance, specific suggestions may also be seen as a preventative measure as well as a treatment technique. This level of assistance obviously requires more experience than the preceding levels, and it is not within the province of the chapter to cover specific suggestions applicable to the many problems that adolescents may present. However, the interested reader can find a detailed description of the application of such suggestions to common sexual problems elsewhere (Annon, 1976).

INTENSIVE THERAPY

It is not within the scope of this chapter to describe or even to attempt to outline an intensive therapy approach to the treatment of sexual problems. For readers who have already received training within a particular discipline and framework for intensive therapy, this is the appropriate time to initiate such treatment. For clinicians who are interested in a social learning approach to the intensive treatment of sexual problems, refer to Annon, 1975.

This concludes the presentation of the P-LI-SS-IT model. The possible advantages of employing this model have been described earlier. It is hoped that the model may provide a framework with which you can continue to develop and expand your knowledge, experience, and skills.

You will naturally have to adapt your use of the model to your particular setting, the amount of the time that you have available, and to your particular level of competence. It should also be emphasized that while the brief therapy part of the model is not intended to resolve all sexual problems, it may handle many.

REFERENCES

Annon, J. S. *The behavioral treatment of sexual problems: Intensive therapy* Honolulu: Enabling Systems, Inc., P. O. Box 2813, Honolulu 96803, 1975.

Annon, J. S. *The behavioral treatment of sexual problems: Brief therapy.* New York: Harper & Row, 1976a.

Annon, J. S. The PLISSIT model: A proposed conceptual scheme for the behavioral treatment of sexual problems. *Journal of Sex Education and Therapy*, 1976b, 2(1); 1-15. (Also in J. Fisher & H. L. Gochros (Eds.), *A handbook of behavior therapy with sexual problems (Vol. 1): General procedures.* New York: Pergamon Press, 1977.

Annon, J. S., & Robinson, C. H. *The PLISSIT approach to sex therapy.* Tape cassette E-7 AASECT, 5010 Wisconsin Ave., N.W., Washington, D.C. 20016, 1977.

Annon, J. S., & Robinson, C. H. The use of vicarious learning in the treatment of sexual concerns. In J. LoPiccolo & L. LoPiccolo (Eds.), *Handbook of sex therapy.* New York: Plenum Press, 1978.

Annon, J. S., & Robinson, C. H. The behavioral treatment of sexual dysfunctions. In A. Sha'Ked (Ed.), *Human sexuality in rehabilitation medicine.* Baltimore: Williams & Wilkins, in press a.

Annon, J. S., & Robinson, C. H. Sex therapies — peer and self-counseling. In W. E. Johnson (Ed.), *Sex in life.* New York: William Brown Publishing, in press b.

Annon, J. S., & Robinson, C. H. Sexual disorders. In A. E. Kazdin, A. Bellack, & M. Hersen (Eds.), *New perspectives in abnormal psychology.* New York: Oxford University Press, in press c.

Annon, J. S., & Robinson, C. H. The treatment of sexual disorders. In C. B. Taylor & J. Ferguson (Eds.), *Advances in behavioral medicine.* New York: Spectrum Publications, in press d.

Baker, L. D., & Nagata, F. S. A group approach to the treatment of heterosexual couples with sexual dissatisfactions. *Journal of Sex Education and Therapy,* 1978, 4(1), 15-18.

Croft, H. A. Managing common sexual problems: a multilevel treatment model. *Postgraduate Medicine,* 1976, 60(5); 186-190.

Daniel, R. S. *Methods and materials for the human sexuality and family life professions (Vol. 1): An annotated guide to the audiovisuals.* 1979.

Fisher, J., & Grochros, H. L. (Eds.) *A handbook of behavior therapy with sexual problems (Vol. 1): General Procedures.* New York: Pergamon Press, 1977.

Gochros, H. L. Personal communication, 1978.

Hindle, W. H. The brief management of sexual problems. *In female emotional problems.* Tape cassette, Vol. 25 (12). Audio-Digest Foundation, 1930 Wilshire Blvd., Los Angeles, California, 90057, 1978.

Kelly, G. F. *Sexuality — The human perspective.* Woodbury, New York: Barron's Educational Series, 1979.

King, N. J. *Handbook of human sexuality.* Unpublished manuscript. Preston Institute of Technology, Victoria, Australia, 1977.

Morton, T. L., & Pion, G. A sexual enhancement group for women. *Journal of Sex Education and Therapy,* 1976, 2(1), 35-38.

Pion, R. J., & Annon, J. S. The office management of sexual problems: Brief therapy approaches. *The Journal of Reproductive Medicine,* 1975, 15(4), 127-144.

Chapter Ten

CHANGING DYSFUNCTIONAL SEXUAL BEHAVIOR

JOEL FISCHER AND MIRANDA S. ARNOW

    STAFF in institutions for adolescents — whether the institutions are psychiatric, correctional, or for the retarded — are frequently confronted by a variety of dysfunctional sexual problems in the inmates of these institutions. Unfortunately, staff members are often untrained in effective, efficient, and professionally responsible methods for helping their clients with these problems. Accordingly, this chapter reviews the types of adolescent sexual problem behaviors that might be seen in an institutional setting and presents an overview of behavior therapy procedures available to institutional staff in working with these problem behaviors. Included also are discussions of the necessity for defining problems in behaviorally specific terms, a rationale for using behavior therapy as a mode of intervention, and the value issues surrounding both adolescent sexuality and the use of behavior therapy in dealing with an adolescent's dysfunctional sexual behaviors.

    The purpose of this chapter is to examine various behavior change strategies. However, when behaviors are to be changed, complex value issues come into play, especially when dealing with sexuality, and particularly when dealing with adolescent sexuality. Our society is, in general, uncomfortable with the concept of adolescents as sexual beings. While the media bombards adolescents with implicit and explicit messages to be sexy so as to succeed, to be loved, and to be attractive, parents, churches and synagogues, teachers, and even peers frown upon an adolescent's sexual explorations. This is indeed a confusing message for adolescents, and for those who are in a helping role. For instance, given our society's present climate of increasing acceptance of premarital sex and the rights of women, a therapist would certainly have serious doubts about changing the behavior of a twenty-three year old woman who is enjoying intercourse with her lover. However, the same therapist might easily consider changing the behavior of a sixteen year old girl enjoying the same or even less complex, sexual behaviors. The adult man who is focused on pursuing women sexually would perhaps not be viewed as dysfunctional, while the same behavior in an adolescent boy may be. The value issue here is, to whom is the behavior a problem, and how great is people's discomfort with adolescent sexuality?

The kinds of sexual problems discussed in this chapter are those which are viewed as maladaptive. The ethical issue, however, is whether practitioners have the right to make the ultimate decision as to what is maladaptive behavior and what behaviors ought to be changed. It is generally accepted, for instance, that many adolescent girls are institutionalized, often with a diagnosis of "adjustment reaction to adolescence," because they have been engaging in intercourse (Ginsberg, 1977) or, probably as often, because parents or physicians are *fearful* that they are (or will be) engaging in such behavior. Or, perhaps an adolescent is viewed as needing institutionalization because he or she privately masturbates frequently. The value issues involved here are many: Who is disturbed by the behavior? Is the adolescent harming anyone, or himself/herself, by masturbating? Is masturbation a viable outlet for sexual expression? Can it be a valid alternative to sexual intercourse?

In looking at the maladaptive behaviors described in this chapter — such as public masturbation, public exposure of genitals, sexual involvement with small children, etc. — the same ethical issues are involved. Is anyone harmed by the behavior? Who is defining the behavior as dysfunctional? Is it ethical to allow an adolescent to engage in sexual behaviors that will frighten others and inevitably land him or her continually in institutional settings?

Attitudes towards sexuality, and adolescent sexuality especially, vary greatly across time, people, religions, parts of the world, and even parts of the same country. Thus far more feasible reasons for changing adolescent sexual behavior pivot on whether the adolescent desires a change, or whether the behavior is harmful to others or leads to incarceration or institutionalization of the adolescent. Still, the value issue remains of defining for whom the behavior is a problem. The costs of changing unwanted behavior in these cases must be weighed against the benefits to society and, much more important, to the growth, self-esteem, and adequate functioning of the adolescent. Certainly a complex value issue involves a behavior where the reaction of society, family, or peers to the adolescent is derision or ridicule (such as an adolescent girl's self-stimulation by rubbing against a chair), even when the behavior is not harmful in and of itself.

While this chapter will focus on techniques for changing unwanted sexual behaviors, keeping in mind the value issues involved, other chapters in this text deal with behaviors that are not exclusively "undesirable." Further, while sex education is an extremely important aspect in both facilitating behavior change and working with an adolescent population, this topic is also elsewhere in the text. It should be stressed, however, that sexuality, responsible decision making, birth control, anatomy, and body image, are crucial educational issues in dealing with adolescents in any population. This is particularly so with institutionalized adolescents, who are generally oversupervised and overprotected from peer discussions of sexuality and from day to day contacts with opposite-sex peers.* Without this sort of education, institutionalized adolescents cannot be expected to learn a repertoire of desirable sexual behaviors, knowledge, and responsibilities with which they can return to the outside world, nor will they be well equipped to fully understand their own bodies, feelings, thoughts, and desires.

---

* See Rosen, 1970, and Edgerton and Dingman, 1964, for some innovative methods for handling this situation.

ADOLESCENT SEXUAL PROBLEMS IN INSTITUTIONS

As with any behaviors that are amenable to change, sexual behaviors often become more manageable to staff and clinicians when they are defined and described in clear terms. When defining sexual behaviors, it is of critical importance to avoid labels. Behaviors, rather than being normal or abnormal, as defined by one or another value system, are best defined as either adaptive or maladaptive to the individuals who perform them (Fischer and Gochros, 1977). If professionals define an adolescent boy as deviant or a fetishist, not only will the practitioner begin to bias him or herself by viewing the adolescent as such, but the client may begin to view himself at that specific label, may well begin to fulfill the negative expectations that this label generates, and thus be perceived by others as deviant or fetishistic. Labeling can also lead people to believe that the adolescent's entire range of behaviors, feelings, and attitudes are linked with that label. If a girl is labeled a lesbian, rather than regarded as a person simply preferring same-sex sexual behaviors, those practitioners who come into contact with her may begin to view all of her behaviors, problematic or not, as somehow linked with her homosexuality. Professionals then may begin to view her simply in terms of that label and ignore or entirely miss other problems she may be experiencing. Labels also imply that the problematic behaviors are concrete entities within the individual and that this individual is always acting, thinking, and feeling as a lesbian, when in all likelihood her sexual or romantic orientation has little to do with her value system, her interests, or her attitudes.

Beyond the danger of the clinician's judgment being impaired by the label so that he or she cannot see anything beyond it, the most critical danger is that the client may come to describe and define himself or herself totally within the context of that label. The "lesbian" may decide that to live up to the role expectations that the label connotes, she must learn to act, live, and behave in a manner expressive of being a lesbian, such as sterotypical mannish (butch) dressing. The inherent problem is that when a client is labeled, he or she will come to define himself or herself as that label (I am a sexual deviant; I am a homosexual) rather than simply defining one of many behaviors he or she exhibits in the course of his or her life. Labels further imply a disease process within the individual and are at best vague and meaningless when considering all the behaviors an individual exhibits across life situations.

Labeling, or defining the entire spectrum of an individual's behavior based on the evaluation of one or two problem behaviors, can jeopardize both the clinician's objectivity and the client's self-image. Because labels are inherently so hazardous, it is always preferable to use definitions of behvaior that are *behaviorally specific*. For instance, if an adolescent girl is labeled as promiscuous, what does this imply? Depending on the definition, and the context of the behavior, the behaviorally specific definition could be that she has sexual intercourse with one boyfriend, that she has intercourse with several male acquaintances, or that she is completely indiscriminate in her choice of male sexual partners. Rather than totally defining an individual in terms of one problem behavior, the use of behaviorally specific terms is far more efficient and accurate in terms of behavior change. When using behaviorally specific terms to describe a behavior, the clinician can more easily focus directly on the behavior that is the object of change. Labeling, on the other hand, could lead to a confusion between the actual behavior and the clinician's focusing on an, at best, elusive and vague disease process somehow inherent within the individual. Using a behaviorally specific term to define a problem behavior allows the clinician to focus directly on the particular behavior he or she wishes to change, rather than on an undefined and broad spectrum of vague problems.

TYPES OF PROBLEM SEXUAL BEHAVIORS

When specifically defining what is meant as a problem behavior, it is important to note that adolescent sexual behaviors may easily be seen as problematic, whether they are harmful or not. Commonly, aside from the discomfort with which some people view adolescent sexuality, there are whole ranges of situations in institutions where behavior that disrupts, distracts, defies, or produces ridicule may be seen as problematic. Whether or not these types of behavior need changing is a subjective, value-laden issue. It is also important to realize that adolescent sexual problems are very similar, if not identical to, adult sexual problems. The only real differences lie in that the behaviors occur in different contexts in relation to age, relative "power," socioeconomic status, dependency status, or peer group within society. For instance, the inability to achieve or maintain an erection is just as much a problem for the adolescent boy as it is for the adult male.* While keeping in mind that not all problematic behaviors are necessarily harmful, and that adolescent sexual behavior is more similar than different from adult sexual behavior, there are certain behaviors singled out for which the techniques reviewed in this chapter might be particularly helpful. These behaviors are probably those most commonly seen in institutions and possibly the most troublesome to institutional staff, but they do not represent an exhaustive listing.+

Indiscriminate Choice of Sexual Partners

Indiscriminate choice of sexual partners is often labeled as promiscuity, and, interestingly, is a term almost exclusively used to define the sexual behavior of girls or women (Arnow, 1977). In the context of adolescent sexuality, indiscriminate choice is often a concern for caretakers of retarded girls, who may lack the necessary judgment as to with whom to become sexually involved. The term implies the inability to make sound decisions regarding a girl's sexual partners and, most commonly, also implies the tendency to have sexual contact with too many partners (although, as discussed earlier, the meaning of "too many" can vary with the particular context of the behavior, and it implies some value judgment). Indiscriminate choice of sexual partners can cause concern when the adolescent girl frequently contracts sexually transmitted disease, consistently becomes pregnant, or when there is reason to fear that her choice of sexual partners is so indiscriminate that the potential for physical and sexual abuse by one of these partners is great (Anant, 1968).

---

* See Chilman, 1978, for an excellent review of the empirical literature on adolescent sexuality.
+ See Miller, 1973, for a more complete review of problem sexual behaviors in the adolescent.

Exposing Genitals in Public

This behavior is usually labeled as exhibitionism, and the behavior is usually limited to males (Fischer and Gochros, 1977; Katchadourian and Lunde, 1975). Katchadourian and Lunde (1975) make the observation that female exhibitionism is much more acceptable, e.g. striptease artists, topless waitresses, than male. The adolescent's exposure of his genitals in public usually involves obtaining sexual excitement from the display of the penis (and testicles) to women (and/or children) who are strangers and who do not expect the display. The inherent gratification of the display stems from the shock and discomfort of the observer (Katchadourian and Lunde, 1975). This type of behavior in the adolescent is problematic because it is frightening to others, shows a high rate of recidivism (Gebhard et al., 1965), and may well be a factor in continuous incarceration of an adolescent.

Masturbating in Public

This behavior may be closely tied to exposing genitals in public, with the same gratification and inherent problems. However, public masturbation may also pose a problem when the adolescent is minimally aware or totally unaware that the behavior is occurring or that it is a problem. (See the case study at the conclusion of this chapter.) Besides being frightening or disturbing to others, the behavior may incur derision and ridicule from peers, family members, and from society in general.

Inadequate Heterosexual Social/Dating Skills

For many reasons, perhaps because of lack of familial socialization training, a dearth of exposure to peers, or continuous institutionalization, some adolescents may never have learned adequate social skills in relation to opposite-sex peers. This may be true for any institutionalized adolescent, including the retarded adolescent (Rosen, 1970). The lack of knowledge about appropriate approach behavior can lead to extremely fearful responses to the opposite sex (Rosen, 1970) and may lead to some types of inappropriate behaviors resulting in institutionalization when the behaviors are never learned (Paul, 1969). The social skills lacking may be those as seemingly simple as carrying on a conversation with an opposite-sex peer, or more complex dating behaviors.

AN OVERVIEW OF BEHAVIOR CHANGE PROCEDURES

There are a number of reasons why behavior therapy is particularly suited for work with sexual problems (Fischer and Gochros, 1977). Since most sexual behaviors are learned, they are particularly amenable to being changed through the directed learning experiences that are at the core of behavior therapy. Further, and of utmost importance, behavioral approaches to sexual problems have been found to be generally more effective and efficient than traditional approaches, and behavioral procedures produce fewer negative side effects than other approaches.

Indeed, most sexual behaviors are rather easily pinpointed and counted. Thus, they are especially suited to the measurement and evaluation procedures that accompany the use of behavior therapy. Finally, since this book is addressed in large part to institutional staff, the use of behavior therapy is particularly indicated, since these procedures generally are more easily learned and implemented than procedures advocated by other theoretical orientations. Additionally, it often is the modality of choice when time is at a premium.

Behavioral Assessment

An essential aspect of the behavior therapy approach is the behavioral assessment. Rather than delving inordinately into the historical causes of the behavior, or using elaborate or inferential diagnoses to describe the behavior, a behavioral assessment attempts to define down or understand the client's behavior in behaviorally specific, precise, and concrete terms and to assess the environmental factors that either keep the behaviors in operation or prevent them from occurring. The sole rationale for this assessment is to assist the practitioner in designing a suitable plan of intervention to change the maladaptive behavior. By the use of client self-reports, the clinician facilitates the client's providing an accurate picture of the behavior and the situations in the environment that sustain or suppress it. The practitioner would attempt to find out for whom the behavior is a problem; assist the client in defining the behavior in measurable, understandable, descriptive, and/or concrete terms; try to find out how long the problem has persisted; attempt to discover what was happening in the physical or emotional environment when the behavior began; under what circumstances the behavior occurs; what eventually happens (either positively or negatively) when the behavior occurs that may reinforce the problem behavior; and what kinds of reactions from peers, family, and society the behavior elicits (see Barlow, 1977; Schumacher and Lloyd, 1976).

OVERVIEW OF STRATEGIES

In many applications of behavior therapy, more than one change strategy is used. As undesired (and desired) behaviors are identified by the therapist and client, the therapist must begin to select the best strategies available for behavior change. Therefore, several strategies may be employed to change one specific target behavior, or several strategies may be used to change several behaviors that are all a part of the client's dysfunction. There is a very real paucity of literature available on the use of behavior therapy with adolescent sexual problems, particularly with those in institutions, although a number of procedures have been developed for work with adult sexual problems.* However, the various techniques that have been used to change undesired sexual behaviors in adults, both within and outside of institutions, in large part also seem applicable to adolescent sexual problems within the institutional setting. Given that adolescent sexuality is more similar to than different from adult sexual behavior and that much of human behavior is learned and therefore amenable to change, behavior therapy techniques demonstrated to be successful in changing dysfunctional behavior in adults can be assumed also to be applicable to work with adolescents, with certain modifications of technique to deal perhaps with age-related differences in experience, knowledge, or self-control.

The change strategy to be used depends on what the problem is. Some problems require a strategy that calls for decreasing certain undesired behaviors, such as decreasing responses that are not desired by the adolescent experiencing them or decreasing behav-

---

*For a general overview of these procedures, see Fischer and Gochros, 1977. Also, see LoPiccolo and LoPiccolo, 1978, for procedures that can be used with a range of common sexual problems such as erection and ejaculation problems, as well as orgasmic problems with painful intercourse see Gochros and Fischer, 1980, for a self-help guide to work with these problems.

iors that are clearly harmful to others, e.g. public genital exposure. Other problems require a strategy that requires simply increasing a desired behavior, such as approach behavior to opposite-sex peers. Another problem may require a strategy that calls for reinforcing a behavior that is an alternate, incompatible behavior to the problem behavior, such as performing vigorous physical exercise in place of public masturbation. The fourth possibility is that one behavior may need to be increased and another decreased, as, for example, in the case of an adolescent boy who is sexually attracted to young children. Here the change strategy would involve decreasing his interest in children and increasing his interest in similar-aged individuals.

In general, many of the available behavioral procedures could be categorized as intended to increase desired behaviors or decrease undesired behaviors. Following is a brief review of some of the key techniques available for work with sexual problems. It should be noted that in actual practice these techniques are often combined to form a behavioral package that could be used to implement one of the strategies described above.

INCREASING ADAPTIVE SEXUAL RESPONSES

The behavioral strategy of increasing adaptive or desired sexual responses is often used in conjunction with, or as an alternative to, strategies that decrease an undesired sexual behavior. In many ways, increasing an adaptive response is preferable to decreasing an unwanted behavior in that a strategy for increasing behavior builds on strengths and positives in the client's behavioral repertoire. Increasing an adaptive response, perhaps while concomitantly decreasing a maladaptive one, can also help avoid the negative side effect sometimes inherent in only decreasing a behavior that may be reinforcing to an individual. Rather than leaving that individual with no sexual outlet, a concomitant increase in a more desired response will provide a new, alternative — and more appropriate — mode of sexual expression.

Provision of Information

Many sex-related problems have their origin in misinformation or lack of accurate information (Fischer and Gochros, 1977). For example, an adolescent girl who has not been educated, or has been miseducated about her body, may be fearful and anxious when faced with the onset of menses. She may not have expected menstruation at all or may have been overexposed to notions of menstruation as a curse, as extremely distasteful or disgusting, or as a loss of important body fluids. Realistic reassurance about the functions and normalcy of the menstrual period can be provided, clearly and comfortably, and can eliminate the dysfunctional myths that would lead to later sexual problems.

Modification of Dysfunctional Self-Regulation and Cognitive Restructuring

Closely related to the provision of information is the debunking of the dysfunctional "shoulds" and "musts" that often rigidly regulate many individuals' sexual behavior and prevent present or future satisfying experiences (Fischer and Gochros, 1977). A typical myth is that the adolescent female or male should never masturbate. The informed, empathic therapist can modify such beliefs and help the client get reinforcement from a wider range of satisfying and appropriate sexual behaviors (see Marshall, 1975, for a case example).

Positive Reinforcement and Shaping Desired Behavior

Through the use of positive reinforcement for appropriate sexual responses, the therapist can begin to shape the desired sexual behaviors. A common strategy in the use of reinforcement and shaping with an unwanted sexual behavior is to shape and reinforce an incompatible, alternative, and more appropriate behavior, which ultimately comes to be as rewarding as the unwanted sexual response originally was.*

Social Retraining

Social retraining involves the use of modeling, role playing, instructions, and assertive training to enhance appropriate sexual and social behaviors, especially in teaching adolescents the social skills involved in opposite-sex approach. Adolescents can view

---

* See Wichramasekera, 1968, for the use of shaping and learning theory in the treatment of exhibitionistic behavior; also see Lutzker, 1973, for the use of reinforcement in the control of exhibitionism in a retarded adult; also see Luiselli et al., 1977, for the use of a combination of reinforcement and overcorrection in the treatment of a child's in-class masturbation. Reference is made to positive reinforcement in a case study cited at the end of this chapter.

films or videotapes experiences; can watch the practitioner or staff model such experiences; and can then role play the experiences, with feedback, either in a group or in individual therapy.*

Guided Masturbation or Orgasmic Reconditioning

The object of guided masturbation is to increase sexual responsiveness to appropriate sex objects in adolescent clients who have inappropriate objects of sexual interest, inanimate objects such as shoes or socks, or age-inappropriate objects such as small children or aging individuals. The principle of guided masturbation is to encourage the client to masturbate to his/her current fantasy until she/he reaches the point of imminent orgasm, at which point the adolescent is directed to shift the masturbatory image to the desired object. Over time, the desired object is envisioned farther and farther back along the continuum of masturbation. A boy who could only masturbate about grandmotherly figures would initially be instructed to envision a similar size female in her place just as ejaculation was imminent.+

DECREASING UNDESIRED SEXUAL BEHAVIORS

As previously discussed, some sexual behaviors are considered undesired because they deviate from certain norms of acceptable sexual behavior. When a client's sexual behaviors are considered unacceptable by him/herself and/or those around him or her, the clinician is faced with complex value issues. The clinician must carefully evaluate the undesired behavior in the context of the client's life situation and in light of always-changing societal norms and standards. The clinician will most likely accept the client's choices unless, as discussed, the adolescent's behavior is extremely aversive or harmful to him/herself or others. If, in the objective opinion of the clinician, and hopefully if the client clearly chooses

---

* See Duehn and Mayadas, 1976, for the use of videotapes in assertive training for homosexuals. See Leon and Gambrill, 1973, for an interesting, detailed institutional social retraining program to increase sophistication and confidence in dating behavior in males, which could easily be applied to an adolescent setting.

+ See Marquis, 1970, for a description of the process and for detailed case studies with adults, which could be modified to adolescents. Also see Marshall, 1973, for the use of orgasmic reconditioning with aversion therapy, and Marshall, 1975, for an interesting method for reducing masturbatory guilt in clients who will be using guided masturbation.

this route, the behavior must be decreased, there are several procedures that have proven useful in bringing about changes.

Systematic Desensitization

The goal of systematic desensitization is to reduce anxiety, which can be particularly useful in helping adolescents reduce anxiety in their approach behavior to appropriate opposite-sex partners. The client is first taught relaxation exercises and is then taken (either in imagination or in a real-life situation) through a hierarchy or graduated series of anxiety-provoking scenes. The first rung on the series is always the least anxiety provoking. Once relaxation and comfort are established with the first rung, the therapist takes the client onto the next step in the hierarchy, which will then be more anxiety provoking than the last. The client is never encouraged to proceed to a new level until relaxation and comfort are established with the preceeding level. For example, for an adolescent boy having great difficulty approaching or feeling comfortable with girls, the first stimulus situation might be walking past a girl without stopping, and the final stimulus situation might be holding hands with a girl on a date, or other more intimate behavior.*

Covert Sensitization

Using covert sensitization, the adolescent would be questioned as to the most aversive or disgusting stimuli he or she could imagine, e.g. vomiting all over oneself. The client is trained to imagine a scene involving his or her approach to an inappropriate sexual object. As the scene becomes arousing, and as the client approaches (in his or her imagination) the sexual object, the scene suddenly becomes terrible as he or she switches in imagination to the aversive stimuli. As soon as the client turns away from the object, he or she begins to feel wonderful. For example, a boy who is attracted to young children would imagine approaching the child and suddenly finding the child swarming with hideous maggots. As he imagined running away from the situation he would begin to feel

---

* It is important to note that systematic desensitization can also *increase* a *desired* behavior by reducing the anxiety attached to it; see Barlow, 1973, for a discussion of systematic desensitization (as well as other procedures) in increasing heterosexual responsiveness.

better and better. (See Cautela and Wisocki, 1971, for interesting examples of such aversive scenes.)

Shame Aversion Therapy

This treatment was developed by Serber (1970) initially to treat cross-dressing behavior. This is an especially good technique for treating adolescents who are prone to grabbing or rubbing against strange women, and perhaps for adolescents who expose their genitals publicly. Though shame aversion therapy may seem somewhat ethically questionable, it appears to be effective in treating those behaviors which may lead to repeated institutionalization, and it is a viable option to chemical and electrical aversion therapy. The adolescent, who is used to a fearful or shocked response from his "victim," and whose arousal is strengthened by the element of surprise, is asked to perform his behavior in front of clinicians or staff, who respond in a neutral manner. It is important that the element of shame be present in the adolescent's feelings about the behavior (Serber, 1970). For instance, the adolescent who publicly exposes his genitals to young women might be asked to do so in front of three student nurses, who very casually ignore him. (See Reitz and Keil, 1971, for an extension of shame aversion therapy applied to an adult male.)

Chemical or Electrical Aversion Therapy

In chemical or electrical aversion therapy, a noxious chemical or electric shock is used to "punish" and ultimately extinguish an undesired sexual behavior. For instance, if an adolescent boy is sexually attracted to leather boots, a slide picturing a pair of boots may be projected on a screen, and if the boy proves to be sexually stimulated (perhaps by using measures of penile erection), he is shocked with an apparatus hooked to his forearm. (See MacCulloch et al., 1971, for use of aversion therapy with an adolescent displaying exhibitionistic behavior.) Shock and chemical aversion therapy can cause considerable therapist discomfort and certainly raise some ethical issues, although patients have not expressed great physical distress when the methods have been used (Marks, 1976). These therapies should only be instituted when no other strategy has been effective, where there is no suspected danger of physical or emotional side effects, or where the behavior has such strongly negative implications or consequences that electrical or chemical aversion therapy would be assessed as not being as negative as the problem behavior.*

VALUE ISSUES REGARDING BEHAVIOR THERAPY

As can be seen from the preceeding description of techniques, behavior therapy is a potentially very powerful means of changing problem sexual behavior. With an ever-growing trend in human services toward the notion that clients should be self-actualizing and able to enjoy themselves as individuals, it is a difficult issue to determine whose values are at work when shaping behaviors via behavior therapy. An inherent danger in behavior therapy is that the clinician will seek change in clients that conforms to either the clinician's or society's values rather than the norms of the individual and the mode of his or her life-style. Again, there is the complex issue of deciding whether behavior change to a prevailing societal norm is ethical, and the issue needs to be carefully weighed when the individual's behavior is causing harm to him/herself or to others.

Behavior therapy, however, is far from being a cold and calculating set of methods of behavior change. Basic values implicit in the use of behavior therapy include the belief that every individual in need of treatment ought to be treated by the most efficient, inexpensive, effective, and harmless methods available. Another value of behavior therapy is that the clinician-client relationship must always be completely open and honest; all of the techniques used to change the problem behavior, all of the goals to be reached, must always be clearly defined and explained. There should never be hidden, ill-defined, or secretive agents to the therapy. Behavior therapy should be easily accessible to populations of people across all socioeconomic, class, intelligence, and sophistication levels. The client must participate fully and knowledgeably in the change process, but the therapist must take ultimate responsibility for the use of the therapy techniques. The relationship between client and clinician, while certainly facilitative,

---

* See Wilson and Davison, 1974, for a critical discussion of shock aversion with homosexual behavior; see also Moss et al., 1979, for the use of positive control as an alternative to shock aversion therapy.

should never be allowed to replace the relationships in the client's natural environment.

In any work with adolescents in institutions, difficult value issues are raised regarding the human rights of clients who may not actively seek or desire behavior change. There are value questions inherent in the institutionalization of any human being. "It is perhaps significant, however, that the potential strength of behavior therapy technology as well as the clarity and explicitness of its procedures bring the ethical issues involved in its utilization into sharp focus, whereas the use of less explicit technologies may permit the illusion of self determination for voluntary clients when, in fact, such self-determination does not exist" (Morrow and Gochros, 1970). Thus, it is important to keep in mind that even in the least structured of therapeutic interventions, reinforcement of the client's particular behaviors, whether they are in the direction of the clinician's or society's norms and values, is always possible (Truax, 1966). Nonetheless, one must always keep in mind that a behavior therapy practitioner must not choose behavior change goals simply because he or she feels discomfort about the client's sexual behavior.

EVALUATION OF INTERVENTION

While using the various techniques available to change sexual behaviors, or any behaviors, every clinician and practitioner should evaluate his or her own practice with clients. In this increased era of accountability, with third-party funders, government sources, and the public demanding proof that interventions are working, every practitioner ought to make an effort to empirically demonstrate that his or her methods of practice are, in fact, effective. Beyond the reasons of accountability, systematic evaluation of practice provides an excellent mechanism of feedback to the practitioner as to which interventive modes in his or her repertoire are effective and which are not. Increased use of evaluation of a clinician's own practice can foster new developments and ideas in human services, which can be transmitted to other professionals and to students.

The single system design is one that can be used to achieve these ends (Gingerich, in press; Hersen and Barlow, 1976). In single system research individual clients (rather than groups) are observed, within treatment and over time, and the desired effect is evaluated. If the change in the client's behavior can be shown to be the result of the given intervention, the practitioner can conclude that it was his or her mode of intervention that resulted in the behavior change. An "essential requirement is that there be some variation in treatment during the study so there is a basis for noting concomitant variations between treatment and client change" (Gingerich, 1977, p. 3). One way to vary treatment so as to observe the correlation between the treatment approach and the client's behavioral changes is to observe the target behaviors in the client before treatment is offered, initiate treatment, and then withhold treatment for a while to observe the outcome (Gingerich, 1977), resuming treatment when the changes in behavior can be seen to be related to the implementation and withdrawal of the intervention program (A-B-A-B design).

Whatever the single system design used, it is of utmost importance that the agent of behavior change monitor and evaluate his or her own clinical practice so as to satisfy him/herself that the strategies are efficient and, most important, genuinely effective. The use of formal and rigorous single system evaluation provides an invaluable source of personal feedback to the clinician.

CASE ILLUSTRATION

While it is useful to overview behavior change strategies, it is as important to observe the direct application of behavior therapy to dysfunctional sexual behavior. Particularly important to note in the following case illustration is that the child's teacher, who was not an experienced behavior therapist, was effectively used as the major behavior change agent, and carried out the reinforcement schedule with minimal instruction and with minimal in-person contact with the researchers.

Wagner (1968) discusses the case of an eleven year old girl who "compulsively" masturbated in class. The girl's teacher was concerned because the girl's almost continual masturbation disturbed other students and disrupted the girl's ability to concentrate and learn at even a minimal level. She usually rocked back and forth on the edge of her desk and sometimes used her hand or foot to self-stimulate. Frequently, the girl reached orgasm, and this response was quite clearly visible to those present in the classroom. Upon assessment, the behavior was determined to have occurred within the classroom environment, though not at home, since the first grade. The other students, while no longer visibly upset by her behavior, completely ignored and isolated her.

Positive reinforcement within an operant conditioning model was the behavior therapy strategy used in this case. One of the major concerns within the intervention was whether any positive reinforcement could be as powerful and rewarding as orgasm, although this was regarded as an empirical question, open to the results of the evaluation.

After the positive reinforcement program began, when the subject stopped masturbating for even a short time, the teacher paid special attention to her with a pat on the head or a positive comment. In the morning, when in the past the girl had been masturbating up to four and five times an hour, if she went without masturbating for an hour, she was rewarded with something she greatly enjoyed doing, which was chosen from a comprehensive list of activities the girl liked. In the afternoon, when the girl usually masturbated up to six or seven times an hour, she was rewarded for one-half hour of nonmasturbation. If she completed a full day without masturbating, a note was sent home to her parents; contingent on these notes, her parents chose from a list of special things to do for her. Eventually, the notes were sent home if she completed two full days without masturbating.

After a time, the girl's desk could be moved from the back of the classroom and back to its original spot in the front of the room without continuation of the masturbation behavior. At the end of the school year, and when the next school year began, it was observed that the girl had not resumed her public masturbatory behavior; thus, the behavior therapy strategy was considered successful.

The undesired behavior in this case was in-class masturbation. However, rather than punishing the undesired behavior, the approach was based on strengthening the desired behavior (non-masturbation) through a series of rewards contingent on consistent nonmasturbation.

CONCLUSION

There is a surprising absence of literature on the subject of adolescent sexual problems in institutions, particularly with regard to effective methods of dealing with these problems. This chapter, therefore, has presented an overview of a range of procedures that are available to be used in dealing effectively with such problems. In addition, some of the ethical issues associated with the use of these procedures were also discussed.

It is hoped that this presentation can serve as a catalyst for institutional staff in at least two ways. First, this chapter perhaps can serve to emphasize that many of these adolescents do have sexual problems that should not be ignored or treated with disdain either because the staff are uncomfortable with the problems or view them as secondary to the primary reasons for the adolescent's institutionalization. Second, by presenting an overview of techniques that are available to deal effectively and humanely with these problems, it is hoped that institutional staff will use this chapter as a stimulus to learn more about these procedures and, eventually, to implement them in their practice.

REFERENCES

Anant, Santokh S. "Verbal Aversion Therapy with a Promiscuous Girl: A Case Report," *Psychological Reports,* Vol. 22, 1968, pp. 795-796.

Arnow, Randy S. *Indiscriminate Choice of Sexual Partners in Adolescent Females,* University of Wisconsin-Milwaukee, unpublished manuscript, 1977.

Barlow, David H. "Increasing Heterosexual Responsiveness in the Treatment of Sexual Deviation: A Review of the Clinical and Experimental Evidence," *Behavior Therapy,* Vol. 4, 1973, pp. 655-671.

_____ "Assessment of Sexual Behavior," in Anthony R. Ciminero et al., (ed.), *Handbook of Behavioral Assessment.* New York: Wiley, 1977, pp. 461-508.

Cautela, Joseph R. and Wisocki, Patricia A. "Covert Sensitization for the Treatment of Sexual Deviations," *The Psychological Record,* Vol. 21, 1971, pp. 37-48.

Chilman, Catherine. *Adolescent Sexuality in a Changing American Society.* Washington, D.C.: U.S. Department of Health, Education and Welfare, 1978.

Duehn, Wayne D. and Mayadas, Nazneen S. "The Use of Stimulus/Modeling Videotapes in Assertive Training for Homosexuals," *Journal of Homosexuality,* Vol. 2, 1976.

Edgerton, Robert B. and Dingman, Harvey F. "Good Reasons for Bad Supervision: 'Dating' in a Hospital for the Mentally Retarded," *Psychiatric Quarterly Supplement,* Part 2, 1964, pp. 221-233.

Fischer, Joel and Gochros, Harvey L. *Handbook of Behavior Therapy with Sexual Problems, Volumes I and II.* New York: Pergamon, 1977.

Gebhard, P. H. et al. *Sex Offenders.* New York: Har-Row, 1965.

Gingerich, Wallace J. "Procedure for Evaluating Clinical Practice," *Health and Social Work,* in press.

Ginsberg, Leon H. "The Institutionalized Mentally Disabled," in Harvey L. and Jean S. Gochros (eds.) *The Sexually Oppressed.* New York: Ass. Pr., 1977, pp. 215-225.

Gochros, Harvey L. and Fischer, Joel. *Treat Yourself to a Better Sex Life.* Englewood Cliffs, N.J.: P-H, 1980.

Hersen, Michael and Barlow, David H. *Single Case Experimental Designs: Strategies for Studying Behavior Change.* New York: Pergamon, 1976.

Katchadourian, Herant A. and Lunde, Donald T. *Fundamentals of Human Sexuality.* New York: Holt R & W, 1975.

Leon, Sidney and Gambrill, Eileen D. "Behavior Rehearsal as a Method to Increase Heterosexual Interaction," *Corrective & Social Psychiatry & Journal of Experimental Psychiatry,* Vol. 6, 1975, pp. 27-34.

LoPiccolo, Joseph and LoPiccolo, Leslie (eds.). *Handbook of Sex Therapy.* New York: Plenum Pub., 1978.

Luiselli, James K.; Helfen, Carol S.; Pemberton, Bruce W.; and Reisman, John. "The Elimination of a Child's In-Class Masturbation by Overcorrection and Reinforcement," *Journal of Behavior Therapy and Experimental Psychiatry,* Vol. 8, 1977, pp. 201-204.

Lutzker, John R. "Reinforcement Control of Exhibitionism in a Profoundly Retarded Adult," *Proceedings, 81st Annual Convention, A.P.A.,* 1973, pp. 925-926.

MacCulloch, M.J.; Williams, C.; and Birtles, C.J. "Successful Application of Aversion Therapy to an Adolescent Exhibitionist," *Journal of Behavior Therapy and Experimental Psychiatry,* Vol. 2, 1971, pp. 61-66.

Marks, Issac M. "Management of Sexual Disorders," in Harold Leitenberg (ed.), *Handbook of Behavior Modification and Behavior Therapy.* Englewood Cliffs, N.J.: P-H, 1976, pp. 255-300.

Marquis, John N. "Orgasmic Reconditioning: Changing Sexual Object Choice Through Controlling Masturbation Fantasies," *Journal of Behavior Therapy and Experimental Psychiatry,* Vol. 1, 1970, pp. 263-271.

Marshall, W. L. "The Modification of Sexual Fantasies: A Combined Treatment Approach to the Reduction of Deviant Sexual Behavior," *Behavior Research and Therapy,* Vol. 11, 1973, pp. 557-567.

_____. "Reducing Masturbatory Guilt," *Journal of Behavior Therapy and Experimental Psychiatry,* Vol. 6, 1975, pp. 260-261.

Miller, Derek. "The Treatment of Adolescent Sexual Disturbances," *International Journal of Child Psychotherapy,* Vol. 2, 1973, pp. 93-126.

Morrow, William R. and Gochros, Harvey L. "Misconceptions Regarding Behavior Modification," *Social Science Review*, Vol. 44, 1970, pp. 293-307.

Moss, Gene R.; Rada, Richard T.; and Appel, James B. "Positive Control as an Alternative to Aversion Therapy," *Journal of Behavior Therapy and Experimental Psychiatry*, Vol. 1, 1970, pp. 291-294.

Paul, Gordon. "The Chronic Mental Patient: Current Status – Future Directions," *Psychological Bulletin*, Vol. 71, 1969, pp. 81-94.

Reitz, Willard E. and Keil, William E. "Behavioral Treatment of an Exhibitionist," *Journal of Behavior Therapy and Experimental Psychiatry*, Vol. 2, 1971, pp. 67-69.

Rosen, Marvin. "Conditioning Appropriate Heterosexual Behavior in Mentally and Socially Handicapped Populations," *Training School Bulletin*, Vol. 66, 1970, pp. 172-177.

Schumacher, Sallie and Lloyd, Charles W. "Assessment of Sexual Dysfunction" in Michel Ibersen and Alan S. Bellack (eds.), *Behavioral Assessment: A Practical Handbook*. New York: Pergamon, 1976, pp. 419-436.

Truax, Charles B. "Reinforcement and Non-Reinforcement in Rogerian Psychotherapy," *Journal of Abnormal Psychology*, Vol. 71, 1966, pp. 1-9.

Wagner, Mervyn K. "A Case of Public Masturbation Treated by Operant Conditioning," *Journal of Child Psychology and Psychiatry*, Vol. 9, 1968, pp. 61-65.

Wickramasekera, Ian. "The Application of Learning Theory to the Treatment of a Case of Sexual Exhibitionism," *Psychotherapy: Theory, Research and Practice*, Vol. 5, 1968, pp. 108-112.

Wilson, G. Terence and Davison, Gerald C. "Behavior Therapy and Homosexuality: A Critical Perspective," *Behavior Therapy*, Vol. 5, 1974, pp. 16-28.

Chapter Eleven

INSTITUTIONAL GROUPS AND HUMAN SEXUALITY:
Threatening or Therapeutic?

JOY D. JOHNSON

THE reader may wonder why a book such as this needs an entire chapter on adolescent groups and human sexuality; yet, when one considers the dynamics of adolescence, one wonders if one chapter is enough. Groups are, to most adolescents, one of the most powerful sources of influence that they encounter. Groups can help or hinder, challenge or threaten, support or attack, and be nurturing or extremely withholding.

Perhaps one of the most important reasons to consider using groups to deal with adolescent sexual issues is that groups are *there*. Whether we like it or not, groups are a very important facet of an adolescent's life within an institution. In fact, this has been true in past experiences as well. Let me make a suggestion. Put this book down for a moment, if you will, and think back on your own adolescent experiences. See if you can recall some of the most significant events of your adolescence, positive and negative. My hunch is that most of those experiences you had took place in groups, or revolved around fears or fantasies about being in or out of peer groups. One of the tasks of adolescent development is the working through of feeling "in" or "out." Adolescents frequently judge themselves as human beings based on how they perceive they are viewed by groups of peers.

Adolescence is also the time of change of primary allegiance from one group, the family, to another, peers. Thus, groups become extremely important to adolescents as a source of input of what an acceptable human being is, as support in the rebellion against adult values, and as a transfer point from childhood as the adolescent pulls away from his or her own family group.[1] The importance that the group has for adolescents is emphasized by Ken Heap:

> During adolescence the peer group becomes the major normative referent for its members. Identity and strength are, in a sense, borrowed from the group, and used as a means of liberation from the expectations of continued conformity to the primary reference group of the family. This enables the adolescent to experiment with new behavior, values, clothes and language. Above all, he may establish his separateness from the family. Life revolves around the activities and the maintenance of the peer group. The new reference group may often, in fact, be more controlling, and demand more conformity than the family.... As a probation officer I sat in the office vainly striving to reach a teenage gang member, who — usually very politely — manuevered himself out of all attempts at meaningful communication and contact. All responses were submitted to the "invisible committee" of his reference group, the young men with whom he had grown up, attended school, started work, and committed joint offenses, and who were currently enjoying the benefits of my supervision. His conformity to their expectations (in this case a circumspect non-involvement in treatment) hindered the development of a relationship with me. I gradually experienced the illogic of attempting to influence an individual adolescent, leaving in the waiting room his reference group of other offenders whose possibilities were infinitely greater than mine could ever be.[2]

Groups take on even more significance to adolescents within an institution, yet adolescents may have greater difficulties becoming acceptable members than they had on the outside. If, indeed, groups are such powerful sources of rebellion, support, and testing the waters of adulthood, they become even more important in an institution. Children and adolescents who are institutionalized are removed from their own parents for a variety of reasons, e.g. delinquency, drug abuse, mental illness, and retardation; consequently, the institution itself becomes a parent figure. The adolescent who needs to rebel, then, pushes against the institution instead of other parent figures. That rebellion against the adult within an institution is similar to that against parents, with one important difference. The institution is the parent figure for *all* of the adolescents within the institution, and when those young people band together to rebel, the group becomes more forceful and more powerful than in any one adolescent case. Thus, the need to harness that group power and to channel it in therapeutic, constructive ways becomes crucial, or anarchy resides.[3] The group has more power than any individual member, and much control over its members, and when that strength pushes against the institution, it is keenly felt.

PAST GROUP EXPERIENCES

There is another problem that these young people face that makes groups a very powerful force. Institutionalized adolescents have undoubtedly had past negative experiences, perhaps with their parents, perhaps with their peers, which have created a situation for them that requires institutionalization. Whatever the reason for residential intervention, these young people have had past experiences (or circumstances) that required them to be removed, at least temporarily, from their home situation. Many of these young people have suffered tremendous losses through the years, and being placed in a setting away from home puts them in a tremendous double bind. On the one hand the natural teenage rebellion, the striving toward adulthood, draws them to their peers as models for behavior and support. On the other hand, the impact of the serious losses makes them not only distrustful of adults but also very much in need of them. This need conflict may be very difficult to resolve.

I recently visited a residential setting for emotionally disturbed girls and was struck by the difference between teens in that institution and the young people in a high school I had visited some days earlier. The adolescents in the institution very much wanted and needed my attention and the attention of other adults. Some of the ways they used to gain attention were not appreciated by the adults in attendance, but it was clear that the adolescents needed not only to impress their peers but also to have contact with adults. In the high school, however, the adolescents in the hall seemed oblivious to most of the adults around them. They had their own world, their own manner of speaking and dress, and they seemed merely to tolerate the presence and occasional intrusion of adult figures.

Compared to teens who are not confined, adolescents in institutions are usually much more influenced by, and have more influence on, adults. This holds true for teens in all types of institutions. In correctional facilities, for instance, an adolescent may have a history of losses and then create a situation that causes incarceration. This does not take away his or her struggle with the adult community but rather forces the adolescent out within an extremely controlling and often punitive environment. Is it any wonder, then, that groups of adolescents become so powerful?

ADOLESCENT SEXUAL NEEDS

But what does all this have to do with sexuality? The comments above can relate to all adolescent issues and not just sexuality. The need that adolescents have for groups, and the power that groups have over adolescent behavior, attitudes, and feelings of self-worth, permeate an adolescent's life. Sexuality is an important facet of adolescent development, but unfortunately, this fact is all too often ignored within an institution or is considered only when controls are needed. The trend is often to close our eyes to adolescent sexual needs, hoping that if we don't notice them they will go away. The onset of puberty is the beginning of adolescence, yet for many teens that important physiological beginning also marks the beginning of repressed sexual desires and needs and strong environmental messages that sex is dirty or bad. Developmentally, people's sexual interest in themselves begins at birth and ends at death, with no stopping in between, but adolescence is a time of intense focusing on sexuality. As young people go through biological changes that make it evident that physically they are men and women, and find that they have sexual needs that were heretofore not conscious or as intense, refocusing on sexuality is universal.

These needs are frequently accompanied by feelings of fear, confusion, and guilt about some of the sexual fantasies and actions that take place. When you put a sexually alive, perhaps fearful and guilt-ridden adolescent into an institution, the process of acceptance of this sexuality, and finding appropriate ways to express it, is too often stopped short. These adolescents, then, may band together to act out their sexual curiosity, feelings, and guilt in a variety of ways — most of which are upsetting to staff and administration. Use of sexual language as part of everyday speech, group activities of a sexual nature, and a great deal of kidding around or sexual harassment of peers may be one of the few opportunities teens have to deal with their own feelings.[4]

Findings one's own sexual identity is a very important adolescent developmental task. This is no easy job under the best circumstances. The task is compounded when parents or acceptable role models are not available. Additionally, being in an institution may make it extremely difficult for a teen to feel like a man or woman. Another important developmental task of adolescence is establishing healthy relationships with adolescents of both sexes. In institutions where the opposite sex is not available, the normal, natural sexual needs may take on distorted dimensions.[5] The institution just does not provide an environment that stimulates normal peer growth. Some children may not have the intellectual, conceptual, or emotional capacity (severely retarded or psychotic) to understand what their sexual urges are all about, although they feel very intensely. These young people tend to follow the lead set by their instincts or their peers, which can be either very constructive or destructive.

Sexuality is an important entity, but it is also a form of expression of many other adolescent issues and problems. Sexual showing off or acting out is frequently a form of gaining peer acceptance, of determining how one feels about oneself, or trying to find love, of getting even with controlling parents or child care staff, and a multitude of other dimensions.[4] It is frequently a means used to impress peers, to prove masculinity, feminity, or desirability, or as a form of anger and aggression. think back once again on your own adolescence. Think about yourself and some of your friends. Can you think of some ways that sexuality was used to express some other need, or ways that sexual needs were acted out in a different fashion? This is true for all teenagers, not just the special populations that we are talking about in this case. To sort all of this out in attempts to achieve mature relationships is a very difficult task!

In institutions young people are faced with an even more overwhelming situation. Often the lack of appropriate parent role models, the single-sex nature of many institutions, the power of group contagion, the lack of privacy, controls put upon young people, and the fear of discussing sexual issues lead to greater than usual acting out, or potential acting out, of normal adolescent strivings. Group pressure is very powerful in these situations.

There are many ways that groups can be used to facilitate appropriate sexual expression and help young people avoid behavior that is potentially self-destructive. Programs can be held for staff members to help them develop an increasing comfort in talking with young people about sexual issues; problem-solving sessions concerning sexual incidents that happen within any institution may be held; and discussing sexual concerns of residents in natural subgroups may prove beneficial. Groups can also be formed to help adolescents find more appropriate ways to express their sexual needs. These might take on a wide variety of approaches, from education to treatment.

Every institution develops its own set of expectations and norms, which are passed on from staff to young people and back again. Norms for acceptable behavior, expectations of staff for adolescents and adolescents for staff, and freedom or restriction to discuss sexuality all have a great deal of impact upon sexual acting out. If you are working in an institution, the first place you must look is at the institution itself. What within the system enhances or impedes channels for appropriate sexual expression in your adolescent clients? What openness is there within the institution for staff to discuss together their concerns about adolescent sexual behavior and to explore the sources of their own attitudes? Is there freedom for adolescents in your institution to raise sexual concerns and issues verbally, or must all of them be acted out, individually or in groups? Before groups can be used as a viable tool within an institution, there must be some readiness, in the institution itself, to recognize adolescent sexuality as a viable, significant, and natural part of adolescent development. If this is not the case in your own institution, perhaps you can suggest group training of your staff and administration to help them learn needed information, feel more comfortable with their own sexuality, cope with their own responses to the sexual behavior they see acted out on the units, and to begin to develop a plan for open discussion among the adolescents themselves.

USE OF GROUPS

If there is openness in your institution to discussing sexuality, then the number of ways groups can be used within that system is almost limitless. Working either with formed groups of adolescents with similar concerns or with natural groups that already exist within the institution, you have the challenge to provide group experiences that lead to better coping of each adolescent with his/her own sexuality. These groups might be educational, skill building, support, problem solving, behavioral, or treatment in orientation, but all should lead to an acceptance of the sexuality of the adolescent and help build in appropriate forms of expression. Frequently, institutions have ward or unit meetings for their staff and residents alike. This also may be a place not only to discuss concerns of the staff about adolescent sexual acting out but also to provide a means for appropriate expression.

One viable means of dealing with the sexuality of institutionalized adolescents in groups is through an educational mode. It is amazing to find that many adolescents, including those who are sexually active, have many misconceptions, much misinformation, and much missing information. Providing experiences for young people to learn the facts can be an extremely therapeutic experience and can offer a way to open expressions of deeper feelings and concerns. Indeed, many adolescents feel more comfortable asking educationally oriented questions than they do talking about their sexual feelings and fears. Also, some teens are able to resolve sexual conflicts without ever mentioning that they are dealing with them personally. One girl in an institution asked some questions about abortion laws and the process of abortion. An educational session was held, discussing the termination of pregnancy. Though the staff asked the girl many times about her new interest, she never acknowledged any personal concern. During the course of this educational session, she was able to make a decision about keeping her baby, though no one in the institution knew she was pregnant at the time. Educational groups can be extremely good ways to help young people get information they need, and such groups provide an outlet for open discussion. These may be educationally focused sessions within a general ward framework, e.g. a movie after dinner, followed by a discussion, or you may have special group meetings around a specific kind of sexual issue with your clients. Many sex-segregated institutions are concerned with the incidence of homosexual behavior, and many adolescents in these institutions are very frightened by the sexual feelings they feel toward each other. There are many ways to handle this, one of which is to provide a series of educational experiences about what homosexuality is and what it is not, and the difference between a practicing homosexual and the normal homosexual feelings of adolescents and adults. These groups can emphasize the choice that young people have in their own life-style and can include physical and emotional factual information that might help the group members to make choices for themselves.[6]

SKILL-BUILDING GROUPS

Another type of group that can facilitate helping residents to express their own sexual issues comfortably and find more appropriate means of expression is a skill-building group. These are groups, or parts of an on going group, that are designed to teach young people skills in relating, in caring for themselves, or in coping with the institutional staff. These groups, which are designed to teach a specific skill, are (hopefully) composed of people who want to learn that skill, and are time limited, based on how long it should take for that skill mastery to be attained. In one coed institution, for instance, a group of young adolescent boys were becoming increasingly obnoxious in their attempt to attract the girls on the other unit. They were disrobing, stealing the girls' panties, writing obscene suggestions on the bathroom and the dining room walls, and creating fights as a way of getting attention of the girls. A very observing child care worker formed a group of these boys to teach them how to impress girls and stay out of trouble at the same time, and taught these young men some skills in relating to females, which they had never had an opportunity to learn. As the boys became increasingly able to get positive responses from the girls, destruction on the unit decreased markedly, and the general morale and attitude of the residents were much better. The sexual showing off moved into a coed discussion group about what boys and girls expect of each other, a much more acceptable form of sexual expression.

SUPPORT GROUPS

Sometimes groups can be helpful in supporting teens through their struggle to understand their own sexual feelings. These support groups are frequently accompanied by, or accompany, educational groups. They are groups where young people are encouraged to ask questions, to share their fears and concerns, and to get support from the leader and from each other about those feelings. Perhaps one of the greatest senses of support is knowing that other people have the same fears and feelings as you do. Other young people do not have the ability or interest in discussing their sexual feelings as such, but support groups where individuals can ask questions, can joke with each other about sexuality, and can gradually learn to admit some of their fears and fantasies can be very supportive and helpful. There are, of course, some adolescents who have the capacity to sit down and seriously discuss their sexual feelings and concerns; there are others who do not. For most teenagers, it is the comfort of the staff that sets the tone for this type of support discussion group. Often even extremely threatened young people are quite able to discuss their sexual fears and to ask questions once they find out that it neither makes the adult defensive and angry, nor is it ignored or pushed aside. When sexual questions are not viewed as a way to antagonize or shock but, rather, are greeted by acceptance of each question as valid in and of itself, groups of teenagers learn, from the leader, to give that same acceptance to each other. This can eliminate some of the nasty teasing teens often do to each other. Think for a moment about your own work within the institutions. Do you exude a comfort level in discussing sexuality, which allows residents to approach you with their concerns? If not, think about exposing yourself to some desensitizing course or other vehicle that will help you increase your comfort level.

Problem-solving groups are one of the best ways to help young people cope with their sexuality, and within institutions they can be used in two primary forms. One is in the unit or ward meetings, where sexual incidents are brought up and discussed. Too often someone brings up a sexual incident, it is dealt with, criticism and embarrassment may occur, and then it is dropped, without taking the opportunity to open the door for further discussion. In one residential school for severely retarded children, an incident was brought up where a young man pushed down a female resident, pulled down her panties, and was making "inappropriate advances." This was brought up in the ward meeting directly and discussed, and the inappropriateness of this behavior was explained to all concerned. Then the matter was dropped. We were having refreshments together after the meeting when I noticed a couple of the residents giggling and talking together, so I went over to join them. When they noticed my receptivity, they explained how they knew what Tommy had done was "bad," but that they sometimes wished he would do it to them too. It offered a marvelous chance for us to talk about the naturalness of the sexual feelings that these retarded young people have, and to help them view their sexuality as something that is not bad or dirty or about which they should feel guilty but that needs expression in ways that will not be harmful to them. Problem solving in a milieu setting can provide excellent opportunities to move from a sexual problem that has occurred on the ward — everything from writing slang words in the bathroom, to intercourse between two residents, to a gang harassment of an inmate — to open the channel for exploration and acceptance of the feelings involved, with alternate forms of behavior discussed.

Another type of problem-solving group can be formed around a specific problem that residents are currently facing. One correctional institution, for instance, had eighteen girls who were pregnant. A problem-solving group was formed to help these girls share their fears about being pregnant and institutionalized at the same time, and their concerns about what would happen with their babies after they delivered. This problem-solving group not only dealt with the current problem of being pregnant, and prospective mothers, but also with their concerns about how they had been used by men and how they had ended up pregnant and institutionalized. As they talked together, they found that their tremendous need to be cared for, cared about, and taken care of led them into predicaments that were only self-defeating. They had the very thing they were after. While this kind of insight might have happened in individual treatment, being with a group of people in the same situation facilitated much greater introspection and support as each girl struggled to face her own issues.

TREATMENT GROUPS

In treatment institutions, ongoing treatment groups can help deal with sexual issues. Special groups can be set up to work on specific sexual problems. Also, a sensitive therapist working in an ongoing, regular treatment group will find that sexuality crops up quite regularly as these young people struggle to find themselves. It is impossible for an adolescent to really struggle with his/her own identity without sexuality being a part of the struggle. Whether or not this is discussed in a group depends to a great extent on the institutional attitude toward sexual discussion and the comfort of the clinician. Without the therapist ever saying anything directly, the adolescents pick up his or her acceptance or nonacceptance as well as a readiness or lack of readiness to deal with sexual issues.[4]

Take a moment, if you will, to think about the wide variety of ways that groups are used within the institution to which you work. Is sexuality dealt with in these groups? If so, is it dealt with in a way that supports and enhances continued discussion about sexual attitudes and feelings, or is it more likely to shut down open verbal expression, thus pushing the young people to expressing their feelings in other ways? Make a commitment to yourself now to take at least one of the groups with which you work and to build in a vehicle for open discussion of sexual attitudes and feelings. Are adolescents able to share openly fears and fantasies without ridicule from staff and from each other? Helping to establish constructive norms for open sharing about sexual concerns is one of the most important ingredients in moving away from a punitive, acting-out environment to one with more openness and freedom to discuss. Open discussion encourages more appropriate behavior; it does *not* encourage destructive sexual acting out.

To help groups reach the openness we have been discussing and the support of acceptance of feelings with an expectation of appropriate channeling of drives, several ingredients are necessary. First of all, the group environment must be a safe place to be, both physically and emotionally. Staff and residents must feel free to say what they wish without fear of serious repercussions from staff or peers. Physical and emotional safety is something that these institutionalized young people very much need, yet they may have no reason to trust that it will be there. You may have to make a special effort to build it in. That doesn't mean staff and clients won't confront each other or be direct with each other, but it means that it will be done within a supportive atmosphere that is nonpunitive in nature. Adolescents know if there is caring about them as human beings beneath the confrontation or your expression of anger. Many of them come from homes where they have been both physically and emotionally abused, and too often, groups within institutions perpetuate the process. Helping them learn to be gentle with each other is a group effort that can be extremely helpful in controlling sexual acting out.

A second ingredient that needs to be present in these groups, both in the larger institution and within the group itself, is provision for privacy. Institutions have a very difficult time allowing for privacy because most of them do not have adequate space or time for it. When my own son was a teenager and was upset with current life situations, one of his ways of coping was to go into his room, shut the door, and turn his music up as loud as he could. Somehow that provided a safe environment for him to work out his next plan of action. Most institutions cannot provide that type of privacy, yet most could provide much more privacy than they do. They may be afraid that privacy will increase acting out. However, the opposite is frequently the case. Does your institution provide ways for the residents who need privacy to get it? Even in groups, whether they are educational, problem solving, or therapeutic, young people need privacy.[5] They need permission from the leader, the therapist, and from each other to sometimes withdraw into their own frame of mind and not share what they are dealing with at the time. Privacy needs to be respected, or the group is no longer safe.

Another necessary ingredient for adolescents to begin to discuss some of these delicate issues is that they have to feel that there is going to be something in it for them. People will not openly share about themselves unless they have the hope that they will get something back: perhaps some acceptance, some caring, or some practical suggestions about what to do to try to make things better. Young people do not need these groups to find out what they are doing wrong; they need them to find out what they can do right. That seems to be a very subtle difference, yet it isn't at all. Helping individuals who have strong needs to find appropriate means of expression (through masturbation, reading, sublimation, etc.) and to realize that their sexual fears, desires, and fantasies are not inherently bad is not only very helpful but a necessary step in the striving toward sexual identity.

There is another ingredient that needs to be present in groups, and this may be a surprise to some. Young people need to feel needed. They want to feel not only that they can get something from the group but that they have something to contribute to it.[7] In a residential setting for severely disturbed adolescents, one girl came regularly to meetings and was very helpful in her comments and suggestions to the other group members. Never, however, did she share information about herself. She seemed to get little from the group for herself, yet her behavior improved. She was much less anxious, and her sexual hallucinating diminished markedly. Obviously, not all of this could be attributed to the group, but the girl felt that the group was one of the most important influences on her and that it facilitated many of the changes that took place in the institution. In this instance, helping others was a significant curative factor.

The last thing that has to be present for this type of trusting discussion to take place is that everyone in the group has to know that *someone* cares whether or not he or she is there. Particularly for institutionalized adolescents, who often grow up with a series of losses and rejections, knowing that they are important to someone in the group becomes a crucial factor in their ability and willingness to share openly with each other. As you begin to work with these groups, regardless of the type of group, make sure that each individual is affectively connected with someone else within the group. This will lead to greater sharing and group cohesion.[6]

Hopefully, these suggestions will help you get a start toward use of groups to cope with sexual issues. However, one chapter in a book cannot cover all you need to know to help groups establish constructive rules and norms so that they will function efficiently. Some of you have had past training in groups to which you can add sexual content. Others may choose to take a course in working with groups or do further reading. Whatever you decide to do to enhance your skill in working with groups, you are working with them daily with the skills you now have. Hopefully, this chapter will give you the courage to try to harness the natural power of the groups within the institution to become more gentle and accepting of the sexual issues that arise. As you feel more comfortable in discussing sexual issues with your clients in groups, you will find that sexual issues arise more often and that the adolescents are freer to discuss them with you. As you start working with formed groups, perhaps ones that you especially set up to deal with sexual issues, make the goal specific enough and the group time limited enough so that both you and the young people you work with can feel a sense of success. None of us need more failures; all of us need to feel successful. Some guidelines might be to stick with sexual issues with which you feel some degree of comfort, to have time limited experiences in coping with sexuality in groups until you feel comfortable enough to let them follow their own course, and to have enough structure in the group that you will not fear loss of control. These guidelines will hopefully give you a structure and the courage to bring sexuality into your group in your institution.

REFERENCES

1. Joy Johnson, *Adolescents Help Themselves.* Paper presented at the National Conference on Social Welfare, 1969, p. 8.
2. Ken Heap, *Group Theory for Social Workers* (New York: Pergamon Press, 1977), pp. 71, 72.
3. George H. Weber and Bernard Haberlein, *Residential Treatment of Emotionally Disturbed Children* (New York: Behavioral Publications, 1972), p. 94.
4. Draza Kline and Helen-Mary Forbush Overstreet, *Foster Care of Children* (New York: Columbia University Press, 1972), p. 99.

5. Simon Meyerson (Ed.), *Adolescence and Breakdown* (London: George Allen & Unwin, 1975), p. 42.
6. Joy Johnson, *Use of Groups in Schools* (Washington: University Press of America, 1976), Ch. 11.
7. Irvin Yalom, *The Theory and Practice of Group Psychotherapy* (New York: Basic Books, 1970), Chs. 2 & 3.

ADOLESCENT READING

Eleanor Morrison and Vera Borasage (Eds.), *Human Sexuality: Contemporary Perspectives* (Palo Alto: Mayfield Publishing Co., 1973).

Chapter Twelve

HOMOSEXUALITY AND HOMOSEXUAL BEHAVIOR

RANDAL G. FORRESTER AND JAMES HUGGINS

HOMOSEXUALITY is probably one of the most schizophrenic issues that exists for the institutionalized adolescent today. On one hand the institution actually encourages homosexual behavior; on the other hand, it reflects the scorn of society in condemning homosexual behavior. This "schizophrenic" response by the institution can do little to help the resident through the normally confusing process of sorting out and understanding her or his sexual identity and, in fact, often leaves the resident with scars that may take years to heal or that may never heal.

How has this schizophrenic atmosphere in institutions developed? The answer is complex, but simply stated, we, the public, have placed a demand on the institution to eliminate *any and all* sexual expression within the institution. This, of course, cannot realistically be accomplished in most institutions. The institution is faced with the problem of trying to keep residents from following their natural desires for sexual exploration and intimacy. Since pregnancy is generally seen as the greatest risk of heterosexual activity, that risk must be eliminated. It cannot be eliminated through birth control, since that would be seen as encouraging the activity. The only other option is to eliminate all privacy between males and females, which is usually accomplished through substantial or total segregation. By eliminating the risk of pregnancy through segregation, the institution has guaranteed, and therefore encouraged, that most intercourse within the institution will be homosexual in nature.

There is, however, another problem. The institution cannot officially condone homosexual behavior, so it adopts a series of adaptive responses. First, it condemns homosexual behavior within the institution; second, it denies the amount of homosexual activity that goes on; and third, it protects this denial by giving a clear message to the staff to deal with this problem on their own.

We now have an institution where supposedly, no sex goes on except for occasional homosexual behavior, which is condemned. The reality is that we have an institution where there is little to no heterosexual sex going on (depending on whether there is substantial or total segregation of the sexes) but where a lot of homosexual sex is going on. The staff is supposed to deal with it, which, to most staff, means that they should ignore it as much as possible.

The institution's message to ignore the behavior is delivered loud and clear to the staff. If the administration had wanted them to deal with it in any other way, significant staff training would be provided.

The important thing to note about this series of adaptations to an unreal set of expectations is that the political and management needs of the institution are primary. The needs of the residents and of the staff are really only of secondary concern. It is obvious that the staff and residents are losers. What may not be as obvious is that the institution and its administration are losers too. They lose because, in the final analysis, the institution is not a sinister place run by villans but a primary care facility run by caring people who find themselves trying to adapt to an impossible situation to do what good they can for the residents.

The issue of the public's demand for the elimination of all sexual contact within the institution is clear. However, two realities are apparent: first, this is an absolutely unattainable expectation; second, if it could be attained, it would impede the normal sexual development (and consequently much of the social development) of the adolescents residing in the institution.

For the balance of this discussion, we will focus on four major areas. First, we will look at some of the problems that homosexual behavior causes for the residents as a whole. Second, we will discuss the special effects of these problems on those residents who have defined or ultimately will define themselves as gay. Third, we will discuss some clinical approaches to these problems, which may be taken by an individual staff person. Fourth, we will briefly look at some policy issues for the institution as a whole, which might alleviate some of these problems.

HOMOSEXUAL BEHAVIOR AND THE GENERAL RESIDENT POPULATION

In discussing the problems homosexual behavior causes for residents as a whole, we must remember that there are different kinds of institutional settings and that the degree of any specific problem will vary from one type of institution to another. For the sake of our discussions, we have defined three basic types of institutions: criminal justice institutions (CJIs), shelter institutions (SIs), and institutions for the emotionally disturbed, mentally retarded and/or developmentally disabled (EMDIs). Regardless of the type of institution, however, there do seem to be some fairly consistent problems.

One of the first things that a new resident is likely to experience upon entering an institution is some very strong peer pressure to engage in homosexual behavior either with one other resident or with a group of residents. This will be most likely in a CJI and least likely in an EMDI. The institution is a closed community, and the new resident, especially if she/he is physically attractive, will be a desirable change from a steady diet of the same old faces. The effect of this pressure on the new resident can be traumatic. To complicate this trauma, if a new resident does agree to engage in sexual behavior she/he is viewed as weak or queer; if she/he does not agree, she/he may gain some status by being viewed as not queer or stronger but may also find that the rejection is viewed either as a challenge or a reason for ostracization.

The second and third common problems are that sex is often used to establish dominance or a pecking order within the institution; consequently, forced sex (rape) is not uncommon. If the resident initially acquiesces to the pressure to have sex, he or she is viewed as weak or queer and is established at the bottom of the pecking order. If one resists, however, this may be viewed as a rejection of the mores of the institutional community. The community may respond by rejecting the new member, thus leaving him or her isolated. This is most likely to happen in an SI. The rejection may also be seen as a challenge, and the peer pressure may be increased to the point of physical violence and/or rape. This is more likely to happen in a CJI. In this case, the sexual violence is primarily motivated to establish dominance. Sexual frustration is usually only a secondary motivation. In an EMDI, rape is much more likely to result from sexual frustration.

A fourth problem is sexual identity confusion. Since a great deal of homosexual activity is being carried on by adolescents who are primarily heterosexual, confusion about sexual identity is bound to result. As previously stated, much of this sexual activity is designed to relieve frustration and to establish power, but needs for affection and intimacy are also present. Courting and the establishment of reasonably monogamous relationships is not uncommon. In both female and male CJIs it is quite common for a physically weaker resident to become the girl friend of a physically more powerful resident as a protection against rape. Adolescence is normally a time filled with sexual confusion, and institutionalization may increase this confusion. Residents often have great difficulty resolving their internal conflicts and questions resulting from homosexual activity.

Gender stress is a fifth common problem. Since most of the adolescents in an institution are heterosexual and are forced to resort to homosexual behavior through deprivation, much of their sexual behavior is heterosexually modelled. Homosexual acts are therefore not viewed as really homosexual; rather, the same-sex partner is viewed as a substitute opposite-sex partner. In a male institution, those boys who are used to relieve other boys' sexual frustrations are viewed as substitute girls. This, of course, can cause them to develop significant gender confusion. Because of the sexist nature of our society, there is a difference in female institutions. Since sex is primarily used to establish a pecking order, the young woman who takes the masculine role is at the top of that order. That she attains status in terms of power does not prevent her from experiencing significant gender stress. Because sex will more likely be used to establish dominance in CJIs and SIs, it will also be more likely that gender stress will be experienced in these settings than it will in the EMDIs.

A sixth problem is inappropriate behavior. Since the institutional setting is geared to the tacit acceptance of inappropriate sexual behavior, the learning of appropriate sexual (and consequently social) behavior is impeded. This is most true in the EMDIs because the staff, acknowledging the residents' disabilities, have a tendency to be more tolerant. Adolescents are often extremely confused after leaving the institution, because when they try to establish the same sexual behaviors they had in the institution, they find that the society is considerably less tolerant.

Finally, there is the issue of staff abuse. Sex can be used as a means of control by some abusive staff. A staff person usually has the option of ignoring what is going on or of making an issue of it for a particular resident. Staff may also have the option of protecting or not protecting a resident from rape. Most institutional staff are conscientious, caring people; some are not and horror stories told by other staff and former residents abound, e.g. stories about several staff persons who put two retarded boys in a pen to watch them "go at it," or about the staff person who felt a resident needed punishment and turned her back while several other girls raped her. Some staff persons may have their own sexual identity problems. Unfortunately, the institution often provides a perfect place for them to act out sexually with the residents.

In reviewing these major problems (peer pressure for homosexual behavior, sex as a way to establish dominance, forced sex, i.e. rape, sexual identity confusion, gender stress, inappropriate sexual, i.e. social behavior, and staff abuse) we would like to stress that, of necessity, we have had to generalize. Certainly, all institutions are not the same, and all residents or resident populations are not the same. Nevertheless, most institutions will have elements of these problems to a greater or lesser degree, and most institutional residents will have to cope with these problems to some degree. This coping will be especially difficult for the resident who has identified or will as an adult come to identify her/

himself as gay.

THE INSTITUTIONALIZED GAY ADOLESCENT

It is generally accepted that approximately 10 percent of the adult population is homosexually oriented. We can assume, then, that this same percentage of adolescents will be dealing with the necessary adjustments to their minority sexual preference while in the institution. Although we have stressed that homosexual behavior is quite common in institutions, this generally makes adjustment more difficult rather than less difficult for the gay adolescent.

Because of the schizophrenic nature of the institution's handling of homosexual behavior, a gay adolescent receives mixed messages. Many residents are acting out in a homosexual way, but it is not OK to be homosexual.

Consequently, anyone who acknowledges that he or she is gay or is assumed to be gay because of a sterotypic body build or sterotypic mannerisms may be subject to verbal or physical harassment. Gay adolescents, especially males, find themselves on the bottom of the power pecking order. Rape is frequently used to "put the queer in place."

Staff generally have a double standard in dealing with gay adolescents. It is one thing to act out homosexually because there are no other sexual outlets; it is another thing to actually *be* homosexual. Most staff members simply do not know what to do with an adolescent who is or feels he or she may be gay. Where does this leave the gay adolescent? Alone, confused, and with no where to turn for peer or adult support.

CLINICAL APPROACHES
TO DEALING WITH THESE PROBLEMS

So far, the view of the way homosexual behavior is dealt with in institutions has been dismal. However, the problems are not insurmountable. Until significant policy changes are brought about within the institutional setting to insure a more healthy atmosphere for adolescent sexual development, we must deal with some real stumbling blocks; however, we must begin somewhere. It is our experience that staff have the greatest opportunity to help or hinder an adolescent in dealing with homosexual behavior and/or a homosexual preference.

To be helpful, staff must have —

1. A basic understanding of sexual identity development;
2. A clear and consistent approach to dealing with behavior problems that arise;
3. A knowledge of themselves as sexual beings and a comfort with their own sexuality.

UNDERSTANDING SEXUAL IDENTITY DEVELOPMENT

There really are no hard and fast facts about sexual development in human beings. Our unique physical, intellectual, psychological, and emotional makeup makes it difficult to generalize about human development. Reactions to our environment and to significant others are unique to the individual. Therefore, no one is sure how we develop our sexual identities, whether homosexual or bisexual.

What does seem clear is that human beings have the ability to respond to both sexes and that most people develop a *sexual preference* for one sex over the other. Some people, bisexuals, find both sexes equally or nearly equally attractive.

It also seems clear that most people do not develop an exclusive sexual attraction. An individual who prefers same-sex persons may on occasion find an opposite-sex person sexually attractive. The same holds true for heterosexual persons who occasionally find a same-sex person sexually attractive.

Sexual preferences can be thought of as a continuum from homosexuality to heterosexuality. Most of us probably fit somewhere in between the extreme end points of the continuum, as documented in the pioneering works of Alfred Kinsey. In other words, probably few persons are 100 percent heterosexual or 100 percent homosexual. Therefore, those who define themselves as homosexual or heterosexual are simply identifying which preference comprises the major portion of the continuum. The bisexual is identifying that neither comprises a major portion of the continuum but, rather, that the continuum is more or less divided equally between homosexuality and heterosexuality.

When a person identifies which preference occupies the major portion of his or her continuum, they are also defining that the other preference occupies the minor portion of the continuum. Understanding this concept of a nonexclusive sexual preference is vital in understanding adolescent sexuality. During this development stage, most adolescents experience attractions to both sexes. They quickly learn that it is not OK in our society to be attracted to same-sex persons, so most try to focus their attention on opposite-sex partners. As already explained, this is made much more difficult for the institutionalized adolescent.

Notice in this discussion of the development of sexual preferences that sexual behavior has not been mentioned. We have done this purposely to emphasize the difference between sexual preference and sexual behavior. Usually if one prefers to behave in a certain manner, one does so. However, if one has no opportunity to behave as one prefers or if there are social sanctions against the preferred behavior, then one *may* behave in a contrapreferential way. Thus, an adolescent may have a preference for opposite-sex partners but may engage in homosexual behavior, and vice versa. Sexual behavior may reflect sexual preference, but it also may not, especially in institutions. What does this mean for a staff person who is trying to help an adolescent who is confused about his or her sexual identity?

Be Careful With Labels. An adolescent may be having homosexual relationships and not be homosexual. It is not helpful to place labels such as homosexual, bisexual, or heterosexual on an adolescent. They only serve to confine the adolescent into an identity that may not yet be completely explored or resolved.

Never Diagnose a Sexual Preference. Especially if an adolescent is confused, he or she may ask the question, "Am I gay?" Neither an answer of yes or no is helpful. In the first place, you don't know the answer. Sexual identity needs to be explored and resolved by the adolescent. You can only help in that process if you stay neutral. Too many adult gay people have been told during adolescence that they were not gay and, therefore, had their sexual adjustment retarded. Often this has meant that their identities were not resolved until much later in life, if at all.

You Can't Change a Resident's Preference. Most sexual theorists are convinced through their research and clinical experience that a person's sexual preference becomes set very early in development. After that time, erotic preference will not change dramatically. A person will probably not have a clear understanding of his or her sexual preference until well into puberty. Many people only attain that understanding as adults, and some people never come to a clear understanding. In any case, no adolescent's experience within the institution (including staff intervention) will change her/his basic sexual preference. The only thing that can be affected by the institution is the resident's sexual behavior.

There Is No Emergency. Often an adolescent may feel that it is important to have her/his sexual identity "all figured out." It is important to encourage adolescents who are confused to give themselves time to explore before making decisions about whether they are homosexually or heterosexually oriented. It is important to let them know that to have sexual feelings for both females and males is quite normal and that, in time, as they mature, their sexual preference will become clearer to them. They are still in a time of growth and exploration; they don't have to have it all figured out; there is no emergency. This does not mean that when you are working with an adolescent who is quite clear about her/his sexual identity that you should discount that. It is perfectly possible for an adolescent to be clear about preferences whether or not he or she has had overt sexual experiences. It is important to take this self-knowledge seriously.

Be Careful About Making Judgements Based On Stereotypes. Despite the growing body of research, which has dispelled many of the myths about homosexuality, most people still believe that homosexuals act in a stereotypic manner. Females who have traditionally masculine mannerisms or males who are considered effeminate are often mistakenly believed to be homosexual. In reality, most homosexuals simply do not fit the stereotypes, and a lot of heterosexuals do. The only information we can be certain of from observing an adolescent's stereotypic behavior is simply that the individual is behaving stereotypically. This information tells us nothing about whether or not the adolescent is gay.

A CLEAR AND CONSISTENT APPROACH TO DEALING WITH BEHAVIOR PROBLEMS

As stated at the beginning of this chapter, it is unrealistic to expect that sexual behavior will not go on in the institution. We must also assume that most institutions have rules and policies that prohibit sexual realtions between residents. So, how can a staff person deal with behavior problems that arise? How can a staff person be helpful to the resident while enforcing the rules?

First, it is of utmost importance to be nonjudgemental in your approach. Most of us have been taught to regard homosexual behavior as abhorrent. It is often difficult to get past this feeling when dealing with someone who is engaging in a behavior we find repulsive. You may have been taught to regard homosexual behavior as sick, sinful, or unnatural. Regardless of the judgements that you make about homosexual behavior for yourself, you have no right to inflict these judgements on the residents. If you approach behavior problems judgementally, you will be sure to alienate residents who may desperately want and need to talk to you about their feelings.

If the policy of the institution is that no sex is permitted, then this rule must be enforced for homosexual relationships in the same way it would be for heterosexual relationships. Often, if the institution is coed, hand holding, kissing, and light petting are overlooked by staff as long as such behavior is between girls and boys. The same behavior by same-sex couples is usually dealt with as a behavior problem or (especially in EMDIs) as an indication of maladjustment or pathology. It is important to treat a homosexual infraction of the rules in the same way you would treat a heterosexual infraction of the same rule. Likewise, if a rule is bent or simply not enforced heterosexually, then the same bending or lack of enforcement should apply homosexually.

Your reaction as a staff person will be a model for how the residents will view the situation. Be careful to focus on the behavior because it is an infraction of the rules, not because it is homosexual.

It will be helpful to stress to the residents that the sexual behavior that they are engaging in is OK, it is just not OK within the institution. Often staff may leave residents feeling guilty about engaging in homosexual behavior if the difference between behavior inside and outside of the institution is not made clear.

Appropriate behavior must be stressed. Staff should try to help residents understand that any sexual thought or feeling is OK, but that sexual behavior needs to be considered in light of the possible rewards, punishments, and consequences for themselves and others.

Rape should be dealt with as a violent crime, not just a simple breaking of the rules. All too often, homosexual rape is viewed as an unfortunate consequence of institutional life. We would not generally view heterosexual rape in the same way.

A good rule of thumb in dealing with homosexual behavior is to reverse the situation and ask yourself, "How would I deal with this situation if it were heterosexual rather than homosexual in nature?" You may find that you would indeed deal with a heterosexual situation differently. If that is your conclusion, then you need to reconsider how you are dealing with the present homosexual situation.

BECOME COMFORTABLE WITH YOUR OWN SEXUAL IDENTITY AND SEXUAL FEELINGS

Through our years of experience, we have seen the importance of this over and over again. When one person tries to help another person with a problem or issue relating to sexuality and is not comfortable with her/his own sexuality, failure usually results. The reason is obvious. *When we are uncomfortable, we act uncomfortably.* If we are uncomfortable with our own sexuality and someone asks for our help in dealing with their sexuality, we may verbally say "OK, I'll try to help," but our whole manner of body language says "No, this makes me uncomfortable." The other person senses this and tries to reduce our discomfort by gradually withdrawing from the conversation. This is true for everyone: parents, clergy, social workers, therapists, physicians, youth workers, and houseparents.

To be uncomfortable with our sexuality is no cause for shame. There is little in our society to foster this comfort. The development of comfort takes self-knowledge, and that takes time. Just as we say to residents, we also say to staff who are unclear and uncomfortable with their sexuality, "There is no emergency. Take your time. Whenever a residents calls on you to deal with an issue that makes you uncomfortable, say that you don't feel comfortable in dealing with it and ask the resident to talk to a staff person who you feel will be comfortable."

POLICY ISSUES

This chapter began with a discussion of the schizophrenic manner in which most institutions respond to homosexual behavior. This response will continue unless significant policy changes are made.

Some members of an institution's resident population will have a clear homosexual preference and will need some homosexual social and affectional experience. Some residents will have a clear heterosexual preference and will need some heterosexual social and affectional experience. Still other residents will be unclear about their preferences and may need both homosexual and heterosexual types of experience. The needs of the residents for social and/or affectional experiences will vary from almost nothing to extremely strong. We may or may not be comfortable with the idea, but we know that adolescents outside of the institutions have the opportunity to and often do experiment sexually with one or both sexes. We cannot expect institutionalized adolescents to ignore their sexuality.

Institutions must define reasonable and *attainable* sexual behavior policies and enforce these policies equitably, consistently, and without bias. Reasonableness implies a judgement, and we suggest that this judgement be based on reality rather than prejudice. It is unreasonable to expect that no sex will go on in an institution (especially if we define sex as both affectional and genitally sexual experiences). It is unreasonable to ignore that homosexual behavior will be quite prevelent in segregated institutions.

It seems reasonable, then, to establish policies that allow for privacy among residents and that take into account the basic needs of residents for physical intimacy. It also seems reasonable to establish policies that deal equitably with homosexual and heterosexual behavior.

Policies regarding sexual behavior, however, cannot be established or enforced without the involvement of the residents and staff. Residents need sex education and the opportunity for values clarification regarding sexual issues (especially homosexuality). Not only sexual physiology but sexual feelings and behavior must be discussed. An open discussion of homosexuality, rape, etc., would do much to dispel myths and encourage responsible behavior.

Staff also need information about sexuality and how to handle behavior problems. Homosexual behavior must be dealt with openly among staff so that comfort around this issue can be increased. The more a staff learns about sexuality and the less it becomes a taboo or dirty subject within the institution, the more the residents benefit (and, consequently, the more the institution and its staff benefit).

CONCLUSION

The issues relating to both homosexual behavior and homosexual preference within the institution are inexorably interwined with the broader issue of sexuality within the institution. We have tried, where possible, to untwine them. Much of what you learn from the other chapters will apply analogically to the homosexual resident.

In some ways, however, the way an institution deals with its homosexually oriented residents will be a barometer of how it is dealing with the sexuality of its residents generally. If we go back to that idea that all people have some homosexuality in their preference continuum and that adolescents are often unclear about their preference and, therefore, involved in both homosexual and heterosexual exploration, then it is easy to see how the institution that reacts to homosexuality with scorn and prejudice does a disservice not only to those residents who are or will become clearly self-identified as gay but also to those residents who have homosexuality as a minor preference.

PART IV
SPECIAL POPULATIONS

Chapter Thirteen

SEX IN AN INSTITUTION FOR NEGLECTED AND DEPENDENT CHILDREN:
A Personal Account

DONALD D. BROWN

MY entire childhood was spent in two East Coast institutions – the first twelve years in an urban orphanage, the remainder in a rural boarding school. This chapter will only deal with the latter institution because it had the most profound affect on my sexuality. Looking back from the perspective of a forty-five year old male, my sexuality appears to a be paradox. I was a very naive, extremely shy, and sexually ignorant teenager: now, however, I am a college professor teaching graduate and undergraduate courses in human sexuality, a sex education consultant to public and private agencies and institutions, a sex therapist, and a newspaper columnist dealing with sexual problems.

The following account of my adolescent years in a boarding institution is true, as is the general location, but the name of the school and each person mentioned herein has been changed.

Mohawk School had an ideal setting, 2,700 acres nestled in the foothills of the Berkshire Mountains, surrounded by dairy farms, small towns, and several large estates where gentlemen farmers raised horses. Most of its land was covered with trees – golden maple, paper birch and over 2,000 pines planted by the students.

However, part of the land was cleared, and corn, beets, strawberries, tomatoes, carrots, potatoes, and stringbeans were grown. Apple and peach orchards covered three or four acres. The fruits and vegetables were either packed at the cannery on campus or stored in the root cellars found behind each cottage.

In addition, the school had its own dairy farm with about twenty-five cows, one bull, and two silos supplied with feed raised and harvested by the students. Pigs and chickens were also in abundance. In effect, the school was almost self-sufficient in food.

Mohawk was founded in 1906 as a boarding school for orphans and children from broken homes by an Episcopalian Bishop from New York City. Therefore, religion was considered important, at least by most of the faculty. When I arrived in 1947, all students were required to attend Sunday chapel services, which I found boring and tried to avoid whenever possible. Participation in an evening prayer service once a week and singing in the choir were encouraged.

Financial support came from a small endowment, state and county welfare boards, the state education department, and donations. Mohawk had a board of directors composed primarily of local upper middle- and upper-class social leaders, prominent businessmen, and leading professionals. The ability to raise money through public, private, and corporate appeals was apparently an important variable considered when choosing a headmaster — much like many of our college presidents.

The approximately 200 students at Mohawk, almost equally divided between boys and girls, lived in cottages. There was one cottage for boys and girls up to the age of eight, and separate cottages for each sex grouped by age: nine to twelve, thirteen to fifteen, sixteen to eighteen. Each of the boy's cottages had a husband and wife as houseparents, while either one or two women were in charge of the girls' cottages. The boys lived scattered around the base of a large hill, the girls were on the hilltop, with the chapel, administration building, gym, infirmary, and school buildings in between.

All students were given an individual psychological and intellectual evaluation before they entered Mohawk. Grades one through eight were in one building, while nine through twelve were in the high school. Academic achievement was encouraged at all levels. There was even a big commencement program and diploma awarded when eighth grade was successfully completed. The high school had a classical curriculum with a thorough grounding in the arts and sciences. Written and oral communication skills were emphasized, and most students were encouraged to take three years of Latin.

At the same time, there was a lot of informality. Students could bring their dogs into most classrooms as long as they didn't fight or growl, and occasionally classes were held outdoors when the weather was good and the ground dry.

Most of the faculty lived on campus and were like good utility players in baseball, assuming several roles at the school. The majority of houseparents were also teachers, as was the resident minister. The high school principal was the football coach, while the elementary school principal served in the library as well and took over an occasional class when the regular teacher was sick.

Like any other institution, there were good and poor faculty and staff members. Some of the teachers, especially in science and English, were outstanding, and there were no extremely boring or ineffective instructors. In looking back, I think that the majority really cared about us, always willing to spend extra time when we had academic problems, or listen when we were upset. Some of the really sensitive ones communicated well through touch – a hand on the arm, an arm around the shoulder, or a hug when most needed.

Unlike some other institutions I've visited, there seemed to be a special closeness between the students and faculty at Mohawk. Maybe it was because most of the faculty seemed to enjoy life and saw the humor in many of the crazy adolescent pranks we pulled. For example, one day nine pigs broke out of their pen, which was duly noted by some teachers and students. The principal sent a friend and me to drive them back to the farm. As we passed the gym, we impulsively decided to drive the pigs into the nearby high school building. Jimmy held the door open while I drove them up the steps. Unfortunately, the school had linoleum floors and the pigs couldn't get any traction because of their hard hooves. They would run down the long main hall trying to dodge the teachers attempting to catch them, but end up by either knocking them over or skidding between their legs. It took almost an hour to round up the pigs. During this time most of the students were enjoying the spectacle and our female Latin teacher was doubled over in laughter, as was I. Three students were dispatched to return the pigs to the farm, and the principal, with a stern look on his face, took Jimmy and me into his office. After slamming the door close, he walked over to his desk, looked us in the eyes, and broke out laughing. We were grounded for a week anyway. It's a shame that this empathy didn't extend to sexual activity. Pregnant students or those caught in the act were usually dismissed from Mohawk.

Having come to Mohawk from an orphanage at the age of twelve, I had little difficulty adjusting to the group life-style. At the beginning, some of the older boys tested me, but after several fights I was accepted as one of the guys. My first cottage had a resident population that fluctuated between twenty and twenty-five boys. Most of our talk, feelings, and fantasies centered around sports and sex. We did better in the former than the latter. Sexually, I was very naive and extremely shy around girls. Beginning around the age of eleven or twelve, I had fantastic sexual fantasies and masturbated at least once a day, sometimes in the bathroom, but usually in my bed at night. Unfortunately, we lived in dorms of ten boys with cubicles open to the center aisle, so there was little privacy. Almost all of us would lie on our backs with our knees up and masturbate carefully so as not to squeek the bedsprings, collecting the semen in facial tissue to flush down the toilet in the morning. There were a lot of jokes about jerking off, but no one admitted to participating in this particular activity. Actually, I usually felt somewhat guilty about masturbation, probably becuase a staff member at the orphanage, who was bathing me around the age of five or six, said I had bags under my eyes and, pointing to my penis, asked if I was "playing with that thing." This attitude, that thou shall not play with thy penis, was somehow conveyed verbally and nonverbally at both the orphanage and Mohawk. Fortunately, I enjoyed my orgasms too much to stop. However, I always wondered if there was a connection between the pimples on my face and masturbation. I questioned the failing eyesight in my right eye because of another myth and

Sex in an Institution for Neglected and Dependent Children 171

became ambidextrous in an attempt to correct this situation. It didn't help.

There was no formal sex education at Mohawk. Even in biology the reproductive and excretory systems were omitted when we studied human anatomy and physiology. I was very ignorant. At the age of thirteen, one of my friends, who had a reputation as a real lover, threw a sanitary napkin on my bed. I didn't even know what it was.

However, there was a lot of informal sex education. One of my seventh grade classmates was caught by another student sticking a hot dog up her vagina in the girl's room. Word spread quickly, and she was very embarrassed. I felt sorry for her, but the comments soon died down. This was the first time I realized that girls also had sexual desires.

Near the cannery was an old nineteenth century cemetary with about six graves surrounded by a wooden fence and large old pine trees. During my second year at Mohawk, I was climbing one of the pine trees when an older student and his girl friend walked into the cemetary and ended up making love directly under the tree in which I was perched. I froze with fright because the guy would kill me if he knew I was there, but at the same time I watched the events unfolding below, getting highly aroused before they even finished undressing. I could even hear my own heartbeat. Up to this point I had heard guys brag about getting "some" or tease about sucking "pussy." Prior to this pine tree vigil, I had only a vague idea of what "some" was, and this was the first time I ever saw a "pussy."

The cannery brings back other memories. One older boy defecated in a #10 can, sealed it up, and put a "BEETS" label on it. I later heard that it exploded all over a shelf in one of the girl's cottages. Also, a group of us were canning tomatoes one day when one of the older girls started teasing her boyfriend. There were no faculty members present, so he told his girl friend to cut it out or he would pull her pants down and stick a tomato up her "pussy." She didn't and he did. She laughingly protested and seemed somewhat embarrassed, but she appeared to enjoy it and so did I.

Most people seem to think that homosexuality is more common in boarding institutions than in public schools. However, perhaps because Mohawk was coeducational, I only had two encounters with homosexuality. The first occurred one night when I was around thirteen. I had just taken a shower and was sitting on my bed reading. I was alone in the end cubicle of the empty dorm when the housefather, who was also my math teacher, walked in. He sat down beside me and started talking, gently rubbing my right thigh at the same time. Gradually my bathrobe opened, completely exposing me. He casually remarked that I had a "nice cock." I was still very naive and didn't know what a homosexual was, but I remember thinking this wasn't right, so I excused myself to go to the bathroom. He never approached me again, and I acted as if the whole thing never happened. The second incidence occurred when I was sixteen. Some of my friends said that one of the seniors in the cottage was "queer." One night six of the guys forced him to perform fellatio on them.

As I look back, the behavior of some faculty and staff members reminds me of *Peyton Place*. The headmaster and his wife appeared to be very pious people. She was, but he was a real hypocrite. Once a group of us were in his darkroom with a dim light on. Standing in front of me was a beautiful classmate with a well-developed body. When the headmaster turned the light out we were in complete darkness. I felt someone brush by me and heard my friend gasp. When the light came back on she whispered to me that someone had grabbed her breasts. I thought it was Dr. Henkel, so when the light went out again I moved into a position where only he would be able to bump into me if he tried to touch her again. Sure enough, he did, and made the mistake of saying "Excuse me." He's now the president of a women's college in another state.

Our math teacher left his wife and ran off to Minnesota with one of the cooks, while the son of one of the houseparents came home from the army and was caught making love in the woods with another houseparent's wife. A secretary doubled as the local village prostitute at night while her twelve year old daughter let us know she was available. The secretary was fired when the headmaster found out about her moonlighting, and the daughter became pregnant at thirteen. One of the farmhands was caught out in a field having sexual intercourse with a sheep and was promptly fired by the farm manager. Two weeks later the farm manager's wife went into a closet and blew herself to bits with a shotgun because her husband was having an affair. He later married his girl friend and stayed on at Mohawk another two years. The business manager and his girl friend were pulled naked and unconscious from his parked stationwagon on a local lover's lane. A leaky exhaust system had caused a high carbon monoxide level in the car, and they had apparently passed out right in the middle of making love. The relief nurse, a woman in her late thirties, had a reputation of giving extra tender loving care to any football players who were put in the infirmary. The faculty really had little more privacy than the students. There were always two or three single teachers dating each other, and we usually knew what was happening.

Despite all the extracurricular activity engaged in by the faculty, everything possible was done to discourage sexual activity on the part of the students. All public events were well attended by sharp-eyed faculty, and all possible places for making out were kept in fairly constant surveillance. Dr. Henkel used to get his kicks by trying to catch students in the act, even driving his car into the woods and fields.

The only approved time for dating was from 2:00 to 4:30 on Sunday afternoons. All couples had to sign out and sign in. We always prayed for good weather because the woods offered the only place for privacy. The winters were usually a disaster. One cold Sunday in February a couple broke into the chapel to make out. Unfortunately, they also got into the communion wine, and their noise level rose with their spiritual intake. They were caught making love in front of the altar, thus ending their career at Mohawk.

Apparently there was a lot of sexual activity going on among some of the students (or so they said) but because of my shyness I seldom did more than pet. If a girl liked you, one of her friends would act as a go-between. If the feeling was mutual, you would start going steady. I had several good relationships start this way, but I seldom made any direct sexual advances. I didn't want my girl friend to think I was only out for her body, nor did I know where or how to start. What little bit did happen was usually because the girl encouraged it in one way or another.

My knowledge of human sexuality came as a result of my own efforts, primarily through various experiences and some library research.

At fourteen, I started working on the farm, which helped me to grow up in many ways. Watching the bull and cows mating was an education in itself. The farmhands treated me like an adult, even teaching me how to drive the farm vehicles and tractors, then sending me alone on errands. I felt like a big shot.

One day, while returning from the barn, a girl around my age from one of the nearby estates hitched a ride. She had on a tight cotton shirt, hair down to her waist, and beautiful long legs. I got an instant erection, which she noticed when she got in the jeep. When we got to the grounds of her parents' estate she led me to a nearby stream, and we lay down on the grassy bank. She took my hand and put it under her shorts. Just as she started to unzip my jeans her German shepherd came barking onto the scene, closely followed by her kid brother. She went off to school shortly thereafter, and I never saw her again. However, those few moments were repeated over and over again in my fantasies.

At the age of seventeen I was still a virgin, but I came really close one Sunday morning when I had skipped out of chapel service because I was working on the farm. My girl friend, who I really liked, and I had just gotton all our clothes off for the first time ever when we heard Dr. Henkel's old car coming. We quickly threw our clothes into our vehicle and took off across the fields. After this she was afraid and broke up with me.

Later that year I walked a girl home from a dance at my cottage. We went into the woods near her cottage and were soon naked. I couldn't believe it. We were both turned on and wanted to make love, but she was having her period and held back. She masturbated me to orgasm instead. After that she thought she was my girl friend, but I was afraid of getting her pregnant and didn't want to marry her, so I backed out. The middle-class mores we picked up at Mohawk in those days implied that if you "knocked a girl up" you had to do the honorable thing and marry her.

Contraception was seldom considered, for everything was supposed to be spontaneous. We would occasionally obtain condoms, which were mostly a status symbol because when you put one in your wallet it made a noticeable circle on the side that you casually let your friends see. When we went to town no one would want to buy the condoms. What rubbers we did have were usually used for masturbation anyway, since most of us were still virgins.

Another source of learning was the library. The only books I really enjoyed were about sports or sex, primarily what little sex could be found in romantic novels. Most of my fantasies weren't just sexual, they included a beautiful love relationship that would last forever. There were no books per se about human sexuality, but I did find one entitled *The Egyptian,* which described lovemaking in a sensuous manner. I read all the lovemaking passages two or three times, usually with an erection. In high school I also read the few books we had by Freud. I really enjoyed Margaret Mead's *Coming of Age in Samoa,* which helped me to understand how sexually repressed our culture was by comparison. The librarian, not aware of my real purpose, was pleased that I spent so much time reading. She would certainly have disapproved, for she even cut out any pictures of nude men and women from *National Geographic* — our version of *Playboy.*

Life at Mohawk was very structured. We got up at 6:00 in the morning, went to school from 7:30 to 1:30, worked for the school from 1:30 to 3:00, then had organized team sports practice or special interest groups from 3:00 to 5:30. After supper we had to study for at least one hour. The boys and girls were separated at work except in the cannery after a harvest. Any weekday contact was discouraged. The high school building even had separate entrances at opposite ends for boys and girls, but seniors were allowed to use the front entrance.

Every Friday night we either had a big school pep rally or watched a movie. Some of the students going steady would sit together, and the boy would walk his girl friend to her cottage afterwards, but she had to be in by 10 PM. This gave them about forty-five minutes after the end of the movie.

On one Saturday a month there was usually a dance in one of the cottages. Although most of us were into sports, we appeared awkward and unsure of ourselves on the dance floor. Since there were only one or two boys who could or would fast dance, the girls would get up and dance together. Faculty members were always present, but some of the good ones made themselves scarce.

Although I was still masturbating almost daily and had a lot of romantic and sexual fantasies, athletics probably dominated my high school life. Sports provided a lot of excitement, dismay, laughs, and memories. Because of all these feelings we shared, we were very close and seldom lonely. Perhaps the companionship and sense of belonging we got from each other lessened the need for other sources of emotional satisfaction.

Sometimes sports and sex were combined. The school spirit was usually very high, and we got a lot of support from the faculty and other students — especially the girls, who served as cheerleaders or faithfully packed the stands. Being on a team made it easier to find a girl friend.

Mohawk was a sexually repressive institution. However, I somehow managed to learn a little about human sexuality, mainly through a variety of experiences, and did establish a sexual identity. Even though the faculty and staff did a poor job of sex education, the majority were sensitive and concerned about our welfare. Because of the closeness of the students and the rapport we had with faculty, we hated to leave Mohawk.

IMPACT

In some ways it's relatively easy to measure the impact Mohawk has had on me. Like most of my fellow students, I didn't have enough money to go to college. Along with three friends, I joined the Navy. My Mohawk experience taught me how to beat the group system, so I was able to maintain my individuality and have lots of fun. Half of my four-year enlistment was spent in naval schools, and I would have made petty officer first class in one month if I had stayed in instead of going to college.

Although I got along well with people and had lots of friends, one thing I really wanted was a family of my own. Shortly after entering the Navy I had a whirlwind courtship with a civilian nurse. We got married six weeks later and had four children in the next eleven years. I've always felt a very special love for my children and have tried hard to give them the emotional closeness I felt was missing from my own childhood.

Because of my need for a complete family, I even tracked down my mother from information I had memorized from my file at Mohawk. This led me to my maternal grandparents, brother, sister, and nephew. This need for a family of one's own was evident among most of my friends from Mohawk, both male and female, who also got married within two years of graduation.

I've lost contact with many of my Mohawk classmates over the years, but three of my best male friends and one former girl friend have kept in touch. We all married young, had children, and got divorced between the ages of thirty-six and forty. Also, all of us have remained friendly with our former partner and stayed close to the children. My former wife and I jointly decided that I would have custody of the children while she had unlimited visiting privileges. All but one of these five friends, a male, is not remarried.

For years I kept in touch with four of the Mohawk faculty members who were special to me. I have not returned to the school in the last ten years. My last visit revealed a lot of new, smaller cottages, but there seemed to be little school spirit. The headmaster seemed more interested in raising money and putting up buildings than in helping children.

Mohawk had quite a positive affect on my self-concept. In listening to the problems other people had with their parents, I can now feel much better about my childhood. I realize that some of the surrogate parents I had at the orphanage and Mohawk really cared about me and loved me. The concern and love they gave to me have been extended to my own children and students.

While I was sexually ignorant, repressed, frustrated, and relatively inexperienced as a teenager, it is debatable whether this was a result of my institutional environment or merely a reflection of society's attitude towards human sexuality. I suspect that the two cannot be separated. Most institutions largely dependent on public financial support tend to reflect the prevailing cultural mores and biases.

A real dichotomy still exists in our culture relative to human sexuality. On the one hand, society has tended to deny and repress the sexuality of its young. This is even more evident in residential institutions, which tend to lag behind society anyway. On the other hand, there have been tremendous changes in the patterns of adolescent sexual activity in the past forty years. Kinsey's research from the 1940s indicated that 34 percent of the females and 72 percent of the males had sexual intercourse before the age of twenty, while recent findings indicate that most of the males *and* females will have engaged in sexual intercourse prior to their twentieth birthday.

Because of these changes in sexual behavior, some valid questions are being raised, and must be addressed. Is premarital sexual intercourse invariably detrimental for our young? Since most of our premarital chastity requirements are directed towards females, what are the cultural and political implications? The main question we must address is how can we assist each adolescent to seek and define his or her own sexual identity and develop an individual value system derived from the past but flexible enough to meet the ever-changing future?

My experience as an institutional consultant as well as a resident indicates that improvement in helping adolescents develop a healthy and responsible sexuality can most effectively take place by upgrading the faculty, implementing a sex education curriculum, and increasing the opportunity for privacy.

Even though the majority of faculty members have the best interest of the residents in mind and are cooperative, they are often victims of their own sexually negative cultural indoctrination. People who do not feel good about their own sexuality can hardly be expected to deal effectively with the sexuality of others. Faculty and staff change would be primarily effected through in-service training in both the cognitive and affective domains. The knowledge should increase their confidence when dealing with the topic in the classroom and informal everyday situations, while the affective should help them to understand and appreciate their own sexuality. Then they will be better able to accept and appreciate the sexuality of the adolescents — both gay and straight, virginal and sexually active.

The primary purpose of a sex education curriculum is the development of a positive self-concept. A person has to love himself/herself before he/or she can love others. Since human sexuality is primarily an emotional phenomena, this objective would receive special emphasis so that each student should feel better about being a male or a female.

A complete program of sex education should be geared to stages of physical and emotional maturation. To give adolescents full license for sexual experimentation at too early a developmental level can add burdens they are not yet ready to handle. They should learn when and how to say no when their best interests are at stake. Mohawk, typical of most institutions, had a definite lack of privacy. At the very least, all bedrooms and toilet stalls should have doors. Opportunities for students to socialize or to be alone without constant faculty or staff observation are necessary.

Specific times and places can be set aside for a variety of social interactions. Respect for privacy – among the students and between the students and faculty – can be developed. As a teenager, I think I knew too much about the private lives of the adults on campus. We all need our space.

Sex education can be broken into two primary areas – sex information and sexual experiences. It is the responsibility of the faculty and staff of residential institutions to provide the information and supportive environment so that the experiences can lead to growth and a positive self-concept.

Chapter Fourteen

CORRECTIONAL FACILITIES

Charles A. Glisson

ANY interpretation of adolescent sexuality within correctional institutions must evolve from an understanding of the unique dimensions of the psychosocial environments of "total institutions." Goffman's (1961) vivid descriptions of the mortifications experienced by residents of institutions imposing total control over the behaviors and social relationships of their inmates provide some of the earliest and best examples of the impact of certain human service organizations on their staff and clients. Correctional facilities are the most total of America's contemporary total institutions and are characterized by a breakdown of the barriers that ordinarily separate individuals in their sleep, play, and work (Goffman, 1961). Variations in geographical space, daily activities, and the company of others are severely constrained, resulting in patterns of behavior and social interactions unique to correctional facilities and having unique implications for the development and expression of sexuality among their inmates.

The adaptation of inmates to the constraints imposed by correctional facilities reflects progressive changes in their perspectives of themselves and of significant others both inside and outside the institution. The potential for dramatic change in those perspectives is greatest for an adolescent whose malleable self-concept and tenuous self-confidence are fragile barriers against the constant pressures of formal and informal institutional structures. This chapter examines (a) the dimensions and characteristics of correctional institutions affecting inmates' beliefs about self and others, (b) the inmates' adaptations to correctional institutions, and (c) the implications of those adaptations for understanding and treating the sexual problems of adolescents within correctional institutions.

ORGANIZATIONAL CHARACTERISTICS OF CORRECTIONAL INSTITUTIONS

Correctional institutions are social organizations with unique social structures and processes that prescribe the behaviors and, to some degree, the cognitive and affective functioning of their members. Therefore, behaviors exhibited by individual members (inmates and staff) can be explained to some extent within an organizational context. In fact, any generalizations about inmates or staff of correctional facilities necessarily refer to those behaviors and perceptions which are a function of the organization within which they are observed. To attempt a description, in other words, of adolescents within correctional facilities implicitly accepts the notion that the described thoughts and actions are determined by the facility. The facility is the common denominator of the inmate population. That and their having been adjudicated as law violators are the only characteristics that all the inmate population share without exception (Newcomb, 1978). Certain adolescent sexual behaviors within correctional facilities are presented here as a product of the complex social organization comprising the institution; to understand that behavior one must first have an understanding of the formal and informal social structures found in such facilities.

Reductionistic approaches to describing characteristics of correctional institutions are difficult to avoid. The stereotyped version of prison life has been advanced as much by the social scientist as by the novelist and, as with many stereotypes, contains enough truth to withstand uninformed criticism. The variation between correctional institutions, as a result, has attracted less attention than deserved, and the identification of variables observable across institutions for the purpose of quantifying between-institution variation and its effect on staff and inmates remains in the neophyte stage. Perhaps the earliest rigorous effort to identify the cause and effect of structural differences between juvenile correctional institutions was reported by Street, Vinter, and Perrow (1966), who demonstrated that a wide variety of techniques and structures could be found within a sample of juvenile correctional institutions. The study concluded that the formal organizational structures of the sampled juvenile correctional institutions were dependent upon the interventive techniques assumed to be the most effective and upon the general perspective that the staff had toward the inmates. These structures perpetuated the treatment philosophy and maintained the type and amount of control considered necessary by the institution's administration. Structures ranged from highly centralized and formalized to noncentralized and nonformalized; techniques ranged from those based on fear and punishment to those based on permissiveness and a psychodynamic understanding of the inmates' problems. It seems necessary, then, to premise our discussion of correctional institutions with the explicit goal of identifying the crucial variables assumed to have the most impact upon individual perspectives of self and, as a result, upon the individual's sexuality. It is assumed that these variables would exhibit a range of values over any given sample of correctional institutions.

The concepts of technological subsystem, structural subsystem, and psychosocial subsystem will be incorporated from the contingency model of organization (Kast and Rosenzweig, 1973) as a framework for discussing the dimensions and characteristics of correctional institutions. The technological subsystem of the organization involves the knowledge base, professional training, and techniques used by the institution in its attempts to "change" the incarcerated individual. The structural subsystem is the formal structure of the organization and is comprised of the hierarchy of authority, participation in decision making, procedural specifications, and division of labor described for organizational members in the organization's plan or charter. The psychosocial subsystem includes the informal power structure, social relationships, and attitudes of organizational members, which are affected by the other organizational subsystems and are the most important in determining the personal adaptation patterns to prison life by both staff and inmates.

The three subsystems are complex systems within themselves, and only a cursory description of their intra- and interrelationships is offered here. The description of these subsystems will hopefully contribute to the conceptualization of the social structures and processes that determine certain adaptive patterns observed within the institution. The psychosocial subsystem is a product of the technological and structural subsystems and a key link in understanding the relationship between institutional characteristics and individual behavior. That link provides an insight into the dynamics of inmate sexual relationships, which would be lost in an exclusive concentration on individual inmate characteristics.

Before discussing the psychosocial subsystem, however, the dimensions of the technological and structural subsystems that affect the psychosocial subsystem should be established. The technological and structural subsystems can be conceptualized in terms of worker/client and worker/worker interaction, respectively. The technology of a correctional facility consists of the activities performed by staff in an effort to change the inmate. Technologies used in changing human beings have been described as intensive because feedback from the raw material determines the type and sequence of activities incorporated in the change process (Thompson, 1967). While human service workers tend to choke on applying the term *raw material* to their clients, it is a term generalized from all types of organizations and used as the basis for establishing the *unique* characteristics of human service delivery systems. For example, Hasenfeld and English (1974) present human service technologies as dealing with a heterogeneous raw material about which there is little knowledge, *in comparison with* other types of raw material processed or changed by industrial and business organizations. Therefore, these characteristics of the raw material result in an indeterminant technology, which has low predictability in terms of outcome *when compared with* other technologies designed for other types of raw material. Organizational theorists argue that such raw materials and technologies demand a specific type of structure if effectiveness is to be maximized, one that allows a great deal of discretion and autonomy among line workers who rely on nonroutinized problem-solving methods.

Worker decisions are ideally based upon a sound theoretical framework acquired through professional education rather than on standardization of procedures. This professional model or organization requires coordination through mutual adjustment between workers, rather than through standardization of procedures and activities, and is in sharp contrast to the establishment of organizational control through centralized and formalized organizational structures. In other words, the pattern of worker/worker interaction prescribed by the organization must complete the type of worker/client interaction necessary for the given technology if effectiveness is to be maximized.

It seems apparent, then, that from an organizational perspective, correctional facilities are classic examples of "catch-22" situations. The necessary control of inmate behavior requires centralized and formalized organizational structures, governing worker behavior as well as inmates, while the required technology demands noncentralized and nonformalized structures if it is to be effective. The control, therefore, is necessary because the technology is ineffective, and the technology is ineffective because the control is present. This double bind is expressed in the split personality of many correctional institutions. The professionals, i.e. social workers and psychologists, attempt to operate under one hierarchy of authority while guards and others responsible for security operate under another. In reality, however, these parallel hierarchies reflect the divisions of labor within a single structure, and claim that professionals can exercise discretion in working with clients while client behavior and relationships are tightly controlled cannot be supported. There are two technological subsystems in operation, one geared to therapy and the other geared to security, and the latter must usually take precedence. This dichotomy results in professionals exercising less discretion in correctional facilities than is generally found among their colleagues in other human service organizations.

The "catch-22" relationship between the technological and structural subsystems affects the psychosocial subsystem in organizationally unique ways. Both staff and inmates develop informal power structures, which are made both necessary and possible through the split personality of the institution. Information, privileges, services, and goods (drugs, cigarettes, weapons, and sex) make up the contraband that fuel the informal structures of correctional facilities. What one can provide or have access to in terms of information, privileges, services, or goods determines that person's position in the informal hierarchy of power. A guard may have more informal power than a warden, or an inmate more informal power than a professional. Social relationships reflect the informal power structure, and individuals with the most power have the widest circle of social relationships. In other words, who drinks coffee with whom and who asks advice of whom are important indicators of the informal power of individuals within the organization.

The attitudes of organizational members, both staff and inmates, comprise another dimension of the psychosocial subsystem affected by the "catch-22" nature of correctional facilities. The frustration experienced by professionals charged with changing inmates' behaviors without the formal structural support required for optimal results and the frustration experienced by inmates who find their work, sleep, and play, as well as with whom they share it, prescribed by the institution, contribute to a psychosocial environment characterized by antipathy, lack of motivation, and violence. Both inmates and staff lack the amount of formal power each deems necessary to satisfactorily meet the demands of their respective roles within the institution. To be rehabilitated and to rehabilitate are goals that fade against the institutional goals of control and constraint.

In summary, control and constraint goals are met by the institution at the expense of positive self-perceptions of both staff and inmates. Staff are unable to perceive themselves as therapists, and inmates are unable to see themselves as capable of normal behavior. Because the institutional roles are abhorrent, inmates develop patterns of adaptation to the institution, which affirm positive perceptions of self. The informal power structures and attitudes of organizational members are reflections of efforts to maintain self-images more acceptable than the roles prescribed by the institutions; inmates, in short, must overcome the mortifications of self described by Goffman to establish senses of self-worth within the limits set by the institution. Those limits are constantly tested by the informal power structures, and occasionally by individuals, and that testing is an important indication of the struggle for the survival of self-worth within the institution.

PATTERNS OF ADAPTATION AMONG INMATES

There are both personal and social patterns of adaptation to correctional facilities, which directly determine the development and expression of sexuality among adolescent inmates. Social patterns of adaptation that emerge in all correctional facilities are characterized to some extent by (1) physical intimidation and violence; (2) the existence of an inmate subculture; and (3) the development of rigid role stereotypes to define interpersonal relationships. Personal lines of adaptation have been listed by Goffman as (1) situational withdrawal; (2) intransigence; (3) colonization; and (4) conversion (1961). Individuals, then, survive in a social structure characterized by violence, a dominant subculture, and rigid role stereotypes by following one or more of the four lines of adaptation.

The specific social patterns of adaptation observed in a given institution reflect both characteristics of the psychosocial subsystem and the structural subsystem of that institution. For example, without well-established informal power structure, a viable inmate subculture could not exist. Because the psychosocial subsystem is affected by the structural subsystem, it would be predicted that an institution with a formal organizational structure characterized by control and constraint would have developed complex informal power structures and an active inmate subculture. The amount of frustration and antipathy developed in response to institutional control determines the extent to which physical intimidation and violence characterize staff/client and client/client interactions. Also, rigid role stereotypes, which ostensibly contradict the prescribed roles of the institution, are supported by the informal organizational structure.

While considerable attention has been given to prison violence in media coverage and in creative writing, it has earned less attention from behavioral and social scientists. It remains, however, an outstanding feature of social relationships within correctional facilities, and the adaptative behaviors chosen by individual inmates are molded by that violence (Johnson, 1978). The thoughts, verbal expressions, and nonverbal communication are affected by and project an undercurrent of violence that cannot be ignored by staff or inmates. Basic survival demands that attention be given to possible violent encounters. Informal power structures, sexual relationships, and institutionalized roles are maintained with physical threats, implicit or explicit, and organizational members are easily enmeshed in relationships dominated by intimidation and violence. Violence or the possibility of violence is a constant, dominant theme within correctional facilities, pervading interpersonal relationships and infusing sexual activity with a level of physical abuse found in no other social institution.

The subculture of a correctional facility is perpetuated by the informal power structures developed by inmates in response to the mortifications of self supported by the institution. The subculture becomes the unit of reference for the inmate, creating an identification of self that is in direct contrast with that of the institution. The subculture, in effect, allows the inmate to reject his or her rejectors (Goffman, 1961). As the inmate becomes familiar with the "ins" and "angles" of the subculture, contraband information, services, and goods become available. The inmate gets one up on the institution and the outside world by wheeling and dealing within the limits set by the institution. The prison subculture captures considerable attention and energy from the inmates; as a result, institutions typically allow its existence within some set of boundary behaviors that are rigidly observed by those who have the most informal power and, hence, the most to gain from the existence of the subculture.

To the inmate, the staff and outside world are peopled by "chumps" who can be "run numbers on" by individuals who "know what time it is." Thus, the psychological devastation of being rejected by the outside world is averted through a put down of those who have rejected. The subculture dictates that one is a chump to work for a living, to obey the laws, or to respect the rights of others; to the inmate the world is made up of winners and losers, and the winners get what they want by any means possible outside or inside the institution. It is significant to note that the acquisition of such items as marijuana, sex, or knives is the source of personal respect and esteem within an institution even though each may easily be acquired by anyone outside the institution. The subculture has a unique set of values and norms, many of which exist within the institution, to provide the basis for an affirmation of self otherwise unavailable to the inmate.

While the inmate may relinquish institutional values upon release, the rigid role stereotypes are an exception in that these stereotypes are internalized by inmates and continue to structure their thinking and behaviors after release. While other values and norms of subculture behavior cease to be functional in the real world, the identification of certain stereotypic roles continues to affirm self-worth and structure a hostile social environment in less threatening terms. The role stereotypes are particularly evident in sexual relationships. Within male institutions, the youngest and weakest inmates become "punks," sexual objects that are sodomized or perform fellatio. While an inmate may use a punk for sexual pleasure, the inmate will treat the punk with disdain and use the term derisively in describing other inmates. While sex role identification may be becoming less of a factor in determining adolescent behavior generally (McDonald, 1978), within the prison subculture sex is identified as a relationship between a strong individual and a weak individual, between a dominant and a submissive partner, between, in effect, a man and a woman in the classic, stereotypic sense. Thus, homosexuality is thereby defined in terms that affirm the self-worth of the dominant man in the relationship, making possible participation in a homosexual experience without the loss of manhood, except, of course, for those who are forced to become the submissive partners. This example is typical of the stereotypic thinking found in correctional facilities and will be returned to in the next section.

Personal lines of adaptation, as previously stated, may follow one of four routes. The first, situational withdrawal, is characterized by a curtailment of involvement with all events and individuals in one's immediate presence (Goffman, 1961). This provides an escape from subculture pressures and violence as well as from the formal demands of the institution. The surrounding environment simply ceases to exist for the inmate.

Intransigence, a second line of adaptation, is characterized by a refusal of the inmate to cooperate with staff (Goffman, 1961). An explicit rejection of the institution, however, is usually short-lived as the rejection takes on more subtle forms as described above. Temporary explicit rejection, however, represents a strong affirmation of self and can be interpreted positively in that light. Intransigent behavior is typically the subject of creative writing regarding correctional facilities, and an individual intransigent occasionally develops a hero image among fellow inmates. In reality, however, most intransigent behavior exists at the discretion of the institution, and lines are explicitly drawn that separate acceptable and unacceptable intransigence.

The third line of adaptation, colonization, represents the maximum use of the subculture and informal power within the institution. Colonizers build comfortable, contented lives within the boundaries of the facility by manipulating the existing social system to their own advantage (Goffman, 1961).

The final line of adaptation, conversion, represents the most disdained of the four among inmates. The convert essentially adopts the institutional role and becomes the perfect inmate (Goffman, 1961). Rather than using the inmate subculture, the staff subculture and staff power structures are used for maximum personal benefit. This line of adaptation can provide protection from intimidation by inmates and, of course, can also be used to intimidate.

These possible lines of adaptation provide methods of coping with the violence and power structures (informal and formal) within the institution. As with most models describing human behavior, there is danger of oversimplification. It may be hard to place a particular inmate in any of the four categories, and most inmates assume patterns of behavior that cover more than one category over time. These personal lines of adaptation and social pattens of adaptation do provide guidelines, however, for discussing the sexual problems of adolescent inmates. It is important that adolescent sexuality within correctional facilities be viewed as a subcategory of behavior found within such institutions and that treating sexual problems be approached in that light. Otherwise, sexual behaviors within the institution can easily be misinterpreted when contrasted with those in the outside world. Moreover, interpreting sexual behaviors for the client within the context of an understanding of institutionalized social structures and processes is one important tool for the therapist. The following section interprets specific sexual problems against the patterns of adaptation and the characteristics of correctional institutions previously discussed and offers suggestions and guidelines for intervention.

THE SEXUAL PROBLEMS OF ADOLESCENTS WITHIN CORRECTIONAL INSTITUTIONS

The following description of the sexual atmosphere of adolescent correctional facilities may seem unduly harsh to many professionals working with adolescents. As stated earlier, characteristics of institutions and institutional behaviors are presented with the understanding that they are present in various institutions in various intensities. While a danger exists that the case is overstated in depicting life within such institutions, the dangers of understatement are ultimately more damaging to the development of an accurate appraisal of expressions of sexuality within correctional facilities. The social and personal patterns of adaptation described earlier form the basis for the discussion here and, as with those patterns, the sexual behaviors presented in this discussion can be applied to *some* extent to other types of institutions and inmates, both adult and adolescent, male and female. It is important to note the continued trend toward earlier sexual experience among adolescents in the general population (Hopkins, 1977); this trend is intensified among incarcerated adolescents (Mannarino and Marsh, 1978).

It has been observed that adolescents within correctional facilities emulate their adult counterparts and pass on values and norms to each successive generation. The role models, in other words, that served to guide behaviors resulting in the adolescent's incarceration continue to function, perhaps even more strongly, within the institution. It is important to remember in reading the following analysis that adolescents are usually incarcerated in correctional facilities only after repeated offenses or a serious felony such as armed robbery or murder. The incarcerated adolescent may therefore be accurately depicted as a bit more hard-core than the usual adolescent lawbreaker. While overgeneralization or stereotyping is to be avoided, the particular characteristics of incarcerated adolescents must be kept in mind if the adaptive patterns described here are to be clearly communicated.

Combining the characteristics of adolescence and the characteristics of correctional institutions produces a stifling environment for the development of sexual behaviors and the treatment of sexual problems. At the risk of, again, excessive generalization, this section describes sexual behaviors and problems that develop within a correctional institution in association with the social and personal patterns of adaptation described in the previous section. At the risk of excessive sexism, the sexual behaviors and problems of male inmates will be discussed first, followed by exceptions observed in female inmates. The sexual behaviors and problems are described as part of the psychosocial fabric of a correctional institution under the assumption that any intervention effort must be based upon a thorough understanding of that fabric if any communication is to occur between therapist and client. Such an understanding is essential for the therapist to place behaviors and problems in a realistic perspective because the sexuality of the inmate develops within an environment typified by sex roles foreign to most of us. In this regard it is important to remember that the incarcerated adolescent has only three sexual options during a time when sex drives may be extremely high: masturbation, homosexual behavior, or abstinence.

Adolescence and incarceration individually offer substantial barriers to a productive therapeutic relationship. In each case, some version of "you don't understand me" is in operation. When an adolescent is also incarcerated, the barriers between the client and therapist are geometrically increased. The age, demeanor, and past experiences of the therapist provide little familiar ground with which the incarcerated adolescent may identify or feel comfortable. This is compounded when the problem area is sexual.

Its essential to add immediately, however, that apologies to the inmate for that lack of common experience are not needed and, in fact, are a detriment to the intervention. An honest appraisal of the inmate's role within a rather unique subculture is required of the therapist, but this should not be construed as support for the inmate's frequent assertion: "You don't know 'cause you ain't been there." This has perhaps been the most frequently heard rejoinder to intervention attempts with inmates of all ages. Intervention attempts are efficiently squelched if a therapist engages the argument of whether or not it is important to experience first hand what a client has experienced before any help can be provided. The beginning therapist may engage the argument repeatedly before learning that one simply cannot convince the client with rational argument that lack of such experience is not a detriment to the treatment effort. That experience is the one outstanding characteristic of self that the inmate believes he or she definitely has over the therapist. "I've been there" provides one-upmanship ammunition essential to the inmate's battle for survival of self, and the therapist can only win the argument through effective treatment.

The male inmate subculture provides the adolescent stereotypic explanations of sex roles, which he can easily understand and imitate. The simple dichotomy of strength, aggressiveness, and dominance against weakness, passivity, and submissiveness is entrenched as the behavioral option for the male inmate. In a misguided effort to preserve some small positive vestige of self, the general social stereotypes of the outside world are distilled within the institutional subculture to their most basic characteristics. An ironic embracing of the rejectors' sex role models and the subsequent exaggeration of the differences between those roles represent attempts of the rejected to establish convincingly their sexuality and worth.

These sexual roles within the institution reduce to being the old man or the punk. It is important to note that punk, or other derisive term, is always used to label the submissive sexual partner who assumes the female role in the relationship by offering, or being forced to offer, his anus or mouth as a substitute vagina to the male partner. This derisiveness puts the dominant inmate one up on the submissive inmate and, consequently, one up on women generally. Disdain for women, as well as substitute women, prevails within male inmate subcultures, and the seeds for that disdain are sown in adolescent as well as adult institutions. Women, substitute or otherwise, are designated as sex objects and, as such, explicitly affirm the maleness of the inmate in the dominant role.

Through such sex role stereotypes, an individual can engage in homosexual activity and also preserve his maleness if he is the dominant partner. The desire for a woman is translated within the institution as the desire for an orifice into which one's penis can be inserted, and any feelings associated with warmth, closeness, and emotional intimacy are flouted as womanly. In short, the adolescent inmate must repress any tender, sensitive approaches to sexual behaviors to preserve his "maleness" in a violent subculture that reveres physical intimidation and dominance in sexual as well as social relationships.

The sex roles outlined above evolve from the social patterns of adaptation within correctional facilities. Individual sexual behaviors develop from the personal patterns of adaptation within that social fabric. The inmate who exhibits situational withdrawal characteristics as described earlier eliminates sexual relationships altogether. Situation withdrawal may be accompanied by a loss of sex drive (although not common among adolescents), continuous masturbation, or, in extreme cases, mutilation of genitalia for sexual stimulation. While self-mutilation is frequently symptomatic of psychosis, representing chronic rather than temporary withdrawal, various forms of physical self-destruction are common among adolescent inmates (Johnson, 1978). In either case, withdrawal is a dramatic statement by the inmate regarding lack of self-worth and powerlessness in dealing with the demands of institutional life.

Although intransigence may also be accompanied by self-mutilation, it can generally be interpreted as an affirmation of self; mutilation, in this case, is limited to cuts on arms and legs, or self-inflicted tattoos. The mutilation is more a defiant act for the intransigent than a manisfestation of self-hate, and it may even be interpreted positively as an indication that the adolescent is struggling to retain some sense of self-determination. The aggressiveness of the intransigent is expressed in his social relationships as well as against the institution, and physical intimidation may be used in his sexual relationships as well. On the other hand, inmates have also reported that frequent physical aggression provides a substitute for sexual aggression, and the lack of sexual behavior may therefore characterize some intransigents.

The colonizer within the correctional institution frequently develops long-term sexual relationships within the inmate subculture. Inmates seek the colonizer as a regular sex partner for the protection and material benefits to which he has access. Or, the colonizer may intimidate a new inmate into becoming a sex partner by using the informal power structure. The colonizer obtains sex on demand and deals it along with other contraband materials in the inmate subculture. Sex, for the colonizer, is a commodity to be controlled and traded in amassing informal power within the institution.

The convert, in contrast, is frequently an inmate who has been abused sexually and finds conversion a necessary step to insuring personal safety. Protection from physical and sexual abuse can usually be obtained from staff in return for ideal inmate behavior. The convert is ostracized from the inmate subculture as a result of his cooperation with staff and is labeled by his fellow inmates a snitch or pussy or some other derogatory term. The convert curtails social and sexual relationships with other inmates and frequently replaces them with staff relationships. While the colonizer uses the informal power structure and inmate subculture to his sexual advantage, the convert seeks refuge from that power through alignment with the formal power structure of the institution.

Sexual problems emerge from the inmates' patterns of adaptation as guilt, fear, aversion, dissatisfaction, and violence in sexual behaviors. The physical abuse, homosexual behavior, and sex roles prescribed by the inmate subculture may turn an adolescent off to sex altogether, resulting in an aversion to sexual expression. Participation in homosexual relationships as the dominant or submissive partner may produce a fear of homosexuality in an inmate who identifies himself as heterosexual. The stereotype sex roles result in immature, superficial, "fuck-oriented" relationships, which are dissatisfying to the inmate and, more important, continue to guide his sexual behaviors after release. Homosexual experiences or excessive masturbation produce guilt reactions among adolescents who have learned that either is a deviant expression of sexuality. Also, the stereotyped roles within the inmate subculture contribute to physical abuse of sexual partners after release as well as in the institution. The abuse may result from dissatisfaction with the sexual relationship combined with a fear of homosexuality and/or a need to subjugate one's sexual partner to fully establish one's maleness.

The above problems are particularly devastating to an adolescent developing a sexual identity and learning sexual behaviors and attitudes that are to last a lifetime. The existence of guilt, fear, aversion, dissatisfaction or violence in the adolescent's sexual relationships, however, increases the adolescent's sexual insecurity, thereby making the clinical identification of the problem difficult. An adolescent will not explicitly present a sexual problem to a staff member or therapist. Communication is indirect in the inmate subculture and, while cues may be offered after considerable trust has developed between staff and inmate, a direct statement of the problem would be unusual in any but the closest therapeutic relationships. For this reason, "hooking" the adolescent into a relationship is a necessary first step in the intervention.

In this initial stage, no confrontation or demands are made by the therapist. Rather, the therapist responds to the presenting problem, usually not sexual, by supporting and affirming the inmate's self-worth. (Glasser, 1965, has provided a lucid description of hooking adolescent female inmates.) Generally, rather superficial assessments of the inmate's situation, i.e. family life before incarceration, how and why he was arrested, relationships with staff and inmates, plans after release, are discussed. Until the inmate perceives the therapist as a confidant and friend, confrontation or directness only serves to intimidate and will be met with defensiveness and/or hostility. This means that the therapist must be especially sensitive to cues once they are offered. They must be picked up in a nonthreatening manner and the inmate encouraged to elaborate without direction giving by the therapist.

If the adolescent can be hooked into a relationship followed by some description of the problem, two responses to the description are required regardless of the specific interventive technique selected by the therapist. First, the adolescent must be reassured of his/her normality. Having been rejected by society as unfit, the fear of being abnormal, while never stated, is especially pronounced among incarcerated adolescents. Second, the therapist can translate the problem or experience as that of an adolescent inmate within a correctional institution, and this understanding is important to the adolescent if it is to be placed in some less threatening perspective. The adolescent is frequently not consciously aware of the extreme pressures of incarceration and, while certainly aware that prison is less pleasant than freedom, may not fully understand that his or her experiences are a function of a unique social environment demanding patterns of adaptation atypical of society generally. So, a translation of the problem or experience in those terms can relieve, to some extent, the guilt or fear that the adolescent may have regarding his/her ability to cope with the demands and responsibilities of sexual behavior and sexual relationships in the outside world.

The etiology of homosexual experience within adolescent institutions has been explained in the past as a combination of deprivation and socialization. It is most interesting to note that Propper (1978) failed to find a main effect of deprivation on homosexual experience among 496 female respondents in four female and three coed adolescent correctional institutions. Previous homosexual experience was the only significant predictor of homosexual experience. The rates of reported homosexual experiences ranged from 6 percent to 30 percent in the seven institutions with an overall rate of 17 percent, which Propper believes is a conservative estimate based upon the method of data collection. Obvious problems with the above findings are that adolescents may be reluctant to report homosexual experiences and that those who do report current experiences are most likely to report previous ones.

So far, the emphasis in the description of patterns of adaptation to correctional facilities has been on male subcultures. While most incarcerated individuals are male and it seems that more literature is generally available on male prisoners, there are some distinct differences regarding sex roles, which must be mentioned. While the violence, subculture, and sex stereotypes are also present in the correctional facilities for female adolescents, the sex roles are a bit different. The overtly homosexual female inmate is at the top of the informal hierarchy of authority, while the overtly homosexual male is at the bottom (Rothenberg, 1977). There has been noted, also, a greater amount of tenderness, intimacy, and warmth between female inmate couples than male inmates. An analysis of adolescent girls' kites (notes sent between inmates) revealed an extensive degree of romanticism and love talk between lovers, with little reference to overt sex acts.

A marked difference in sex role identification has been observed among adolescent female inmates, which transcends earlier findings that female adolescents in institutions are less feminine than the norm (Steele, 1971). Mannarino and March (1978) found that two distinct groups could be identified among incarcerated female adolescents. One group, which had been incarcerated for some type of sexual offense or sexual delinquency, was found to be as feminine as the controls, while the other group, which had been arrested for antisocial behavior such as armed robbery or burglary, was found to be significantly more masculine than both the controls and the sexual offenders.

It seems that in the female inmate subculture as well as the male, society's norms are reflected in microcosm. That the male has the most power and that tenderness and expressions of love are condoned between females accurately reflect society's dictates. Because women are generally less fearful of expressions of tenderness and warmth, it might be assumed that less problems related to sexuality might emerge within correctional facilities. This does not seem to be the case, although pitifully little research is available regarding male/female adolescent sexuality in correctional institutions.

Adolescent female inmates are as likely to be dissatisfied with sexual relationships, feel guilty about masturbation and homosexual experiences, and to develop aversions to sexual activity as described earlier. The patterns of adaptation apply to correctional facilities for females as well as males, and those patterns produce similar reactions with the exception of the sex roles described above.

Specific interventive techniques for particular problems are described in other chapters and can be aptly applied to incarcerated adolescents. Before those techniques can be used, the problem has to be shared with the therapist. The therapist, as described earlier, must be able to place the sexual experiences of the inmate within the context of the psychosocial environment of a correctional facility if the inmate is to feel comfortable in sharing his or her experiences and if those experiences are to be meaningfully and usefully interpreted for the inmate by the therapist. For these reasons, a considerable effort has been made to describe fully characteristics of formal and informal structures, the role stereotypes within the inmate subculture, and the social and personal patterns of adaptation that affect sexual behavior and create sexual problems within adolescent correctional facilities. This description hopefully provides information beneficial to therapeutic attempts at eliciting and interpreting the sexual experiences and problems of incarcerated adolescents.

A secondary objective of this chapter has been to call attention to intervention possibilities at the organization level. Preliminary evidence points to a strong relationship between dimensions of organizational structure and dimensions of the treatment effort, or technology, of the organization (Street, Vinter, and Perrow, 1966; Glisson, 1978). If the preceeding model connecting characteristics of correctional facilities with inmate behaviors is a valid one, promising approaches to improving adaptive patterns among inmate populations through the manipulation of system variables have been generally overlooked. While the contradictory objectives of control and treatment present formidable barriers to behavior change, further exploration of these methods is needed. Examples include adjusting formal control over inmate behavior between units, or between facilities, according to the number and type of offenses to segregate first timers from the well-developed informal power structure of inmates with longer histories of incarceration. Another example of system level intervention is the elimination of formalized divisions of labor among staff. Less formalized divisions of labor have been found to contribute to staff perceiving clients as individuals with unique problems demanding individualized treatment approaches in a variety of human services, including correctional facilities (Glisson, 1978). As a result, team approaches to decision making, problem solving, and treatment planning have become increasingly popular in mental health and should be extended in corrections. Until now, investigations of intervention methods have unfortunately exhibited a myopic tendency to concentrate on clinical variables.

In summary, adolescent inmate sexual problems have been presented as a function of individual and group adaptation to a unique type of complex social organization. Successful intervention efforts, whether at the inmate or the system level, are therefore dependent upon the identification of social and personal patterns of adaptation comprising the psychosocial subsystem within which the inmate exists. Those patterns have been fully described and linked to specific sexual behaviors observed among adolescent inmates. An attempt has been made to avoid overgeneralization or stereotyping while pointing out those patterns and problems which consistently emerge in adolescent correctional facilities.

REFERENCES

Glasser, William, *Reality Therapy*, Harper and Row, New York, 1965.
Glisson, Charles, "Dependence of Technological Routinization on Structural Variables in Human Service Organizations," *Administrative Science Quarterly*, 23, 383-395, 1978.
Goffman, Erving, *Asylums*, Doubleday, Garden City, N.Y., 1961.
Hasenfeld, Yeheskel and Richard A. English, *Human Service Organizations*, University of Michigan Press, Ann Arbor, 1974.
Hopkins, J. Roy, "Sexual Behavior in Adolescence," *Journal of Social Issues*, 33(2): 67-85, 1977.
Johnson, Robert, "Youth in Crisis: Dimensions of Self-Destructive Conduct Among Adolescent Prisoners," *Adolescence*, 13(51): 461-482, 1978.
Kast, Fremont E. and James E. Rosenzweig, *Contingency Views of Organization and Management*, Science Research Associates, Chicago, 1973.
Mannarino, Anthony P. and Marion E. Marsh, "The Relationship Between Sex Role Identification and Juvenile Delinquency in Adolescent Girls," *Adolescence*, 13(52): 643-652, 1978.
McDonald, Gerald W., "A Reconsideration of the Concept 'Sex-Role Identification' in Adolescent and Family Research," *Adolescence* 13(50): 215-220, 1978.
Newcomb, Theodore, "Youth in Colleges and in Corrections: Institutional Influences," *American Psychologist*, 33(2): 114-124, 1978.
Propper, Alice M., "Lesbianism in Female and Coed Correctional Institutions," *Journal of Homosexuality*, 3(3): 265-274, 1978.
Rothenberg, David, "Prisoners," in Harvey L. Gochros and Jean S. Gochros (Eds.), *The Sexually Oppressed*, Association Press, New York, 1977.
Steele, C., "Sexual Identity Problems Among Adolescent Girls in Institutional Placement," *Adolescence*, 6: 509-522, 1971.
Street, David, Robert, D. Vinter, and Charles Perrow, "Executiveship in Juvenile Correctional Institutions," *Organizations for Treatment*, Free Press, New York, 1966.
Thompson, James D., *Organizations in Action*, McGraw-Hill, New York, 1967.

Chapter Fifteen

EMOTIONALLY DISTURBED

Delene Iacono-Harris and David A. Iacono-Harris

THIS chapter, while acknowledging the breadth of the term *emotional disturbance,* will address issues of sexuality for adolescents who are institutionalized because of emotional problems. It is *not* the intent of the authors to give specific information on ways to work out acceptable methods of sexual expression for any and all emotional problems. It *is* the intent of the authors to encourage the creation of a certain milieu in institutions, which accepts sexuality as an integral part of every person and views adolescents with emotional problems as sexual beings. It is also the intent of the authors to emphasize the importance of staffs within institutions not only allowing but actively encouraging exploration of the adolescents' sexuality, rather than attempting to suppress it.

There are many reasons why adults deny or try to suppress the sexuality and sexual behavior of adolescents with emotional problems. While none of these reasons may be valid, all are real. The first reason is simply that they *are* adolescents. Generally, in this society, adolescents are threatening to adults. They judge adults and adult society harshly, and this can be intimidating and unsettling. Adults, in turn, attempt to control adolescents, insisting that they grow in the accepted way. This is especially true in the areas of sexuality and sexual behavior.

The second reason for sexual repression is that the adolescents are institutionalized. Institutionalized persons lose many of the things that are generally taken for granted and espoused as rights of individuals. Existing institutions, by and large, do not afford expressions of individuality, nor do they provide for privacy, autonomy, and freedom. There is a prevading feeling that persons have forfeited these individual rights by virtue of entering an institution. Again, the areas of sexuality and sexual behavior are prime examples of this lack of rights.

Finally, sexual repression occurs when adolescents are emotionally disturbed. Whichever way they go in terms of their developing sexuality, their actions will be attributed to their emotional problems. If they *do* express their sexuality, it very likely will be attributed to their emotional instability. If they *do not* express their sexuality, it most likely will be attributed to their emotional immaturity and insecurity in managing close relationships; therefore, they should not be encouraged. However, an overview of the characteristics of adolescence will show that those who are institutionalized with emotional problems differ from noninstitutionalized adolescents mainly in the degree of their problems, not in the problems themselves. As Chapman says in speaking of emotional normality, "the precise point at which 'within normal limits' ends and 'abnormality' begins is often hard to define, frequently subject to debate, and to some extent is influenced by cultural and economic factors."[1]

For most persons in our society, adolescence is a time of turmoil. The developmental tensions creating this upheaval appear to be a normal part of this life stage.[2] These developmental tensions serve to promote the growth of qualities essential to the functioning adult; their importance, therefore, is not to be underplayed. In his/her growth toward independence, the adolescent will sometimes be in conflict with those in authority. Peers are important allies in this struggle, since they are also working toward the same goal of independence. To strengthen this bond, adolescents often adopt mannerisms, styles of dress, and language similar to one another. Because their own sense of self is not very strong during this time, they rely heavily upon the group. While they need to view certain people and situations idealistically, they are much more aware of the possibility of disillusionment than they were during their earlier years. This possibility of disillusionment accounts for many of the protective veneers of adolescence —

skepticism, cynicism, and basic intolerance of hypocrisy.

Concurrent with the developmental tensions *within* the adolescent are the tensions *between* the adolescent and the adult. As noted earlier, the growth in the adolescent's intellectual abilities makes him/her threatening to adults. The physical changes of the adolescent may create sexual tensions for adults. Adults often find the adolescent's sensitivity to the motivations of others disconcerting.

Developmental tensions within the adolescent and between the adolescent and adults make the emotional balance of the adolescent very tenuous. In general, individuals within institutions are often experiencing tensions that fall outside of the usual range of conflict. Not infrequently, these adolescents present management problems to the adults in their immediate environment — home, school, recreational groups, etc. In extremity they can be dangerous to themselves and/or others, or they can be withdrawn and out of contact with reality. For many, the problems have been with them since childhood, and the tensions of adolescence bring the situation to a crisis state. Others "lack the imagination and judgment to make the greatest display of nonconformity with the least actual deviation therefrom."[3] It is important to realize, however, that simply because an adolescent is having problems in one or several areas does not mean that he/she should be denied the experiences needed for the growth and enrichment of one's total personality.

Before discussing the area of sexuality, let us look briefly at what is meant by adolescence, adolescent behavior, adulthood, and maturity. Adolescence is a period of physical, psychological, social, and emotional growth, which takes a person from childhood to adulthood. Every person in our society between ten and twenty-one years of age is an adolescent. Every person in this society becomes an adult somewhere between eighteen and twenty-five years of age. However, adolescence and adulthood do not always suggest behavior and maturity. Adults who act maturely in most areas of their lives exhibit some adolescent behavior; some adults exhibit much of this behavior. Many adolescents act quite maturely; others act as if they will never be truly mature. Indeed, there is developmental tension in every individual, and the mature person is the one who is striving to come to terms with all aspects of his/her self.

If acceptance of one's physical self, attainment of emotional control, achievement of social maturity, and development of intellectual sophistication and sensitivity can, in a broad sense, be considered the developmental tasks of adolescence, then the emotionally disturbed adolescent is experiencing unusual difficulty in one or more of these developmental areas.[4] This difficulty will have an impact on all the developmental areas but will not totally impede them. The same is true for the emotionally disturbed adolescent with regard to sexuality. While sexuality is often a pervasive component of personality throughout one's life, this seems especially true during adolescence. Sexuality can be a cause and a result of emotional problems for both the institutionalized and noninstitutionalized adolescent. However, that it is problematic does not mean that it can or should be ignored. Sexuality, and in many cases sexual behavior, continues to develop and take form, regardless of the obstacles or impediments placed in its path. Emotionally disturbed adolescents are sexual beings who are striving to develop into mature adult sexual beings. Persons working with disturbed adolescents need to be aware of the sexual tensions in adolescents and especially need to be comfortable with the range of their own sexual tensions and responses. A sexually mature adult will be better prepared to help the disturbed adolescent come to grips with his/her own sexuality. It is for this reason that staff training is the core of any human sexuality program for institutionalized emotionally disturbed adolescents.

STAFF TRAINING

The creation of a milieu that encourages the adolescent's exploration of his/her sexuality requires commitment and creativity. It demands a commitment to the rights of emotionally disturbed adolescents as sexual beings and the creativity to structure a supportive milieu of this. One of the primary tasks in creating such an environment is training for *every* staff member. As a result of the taboos this society places on sex, lack of information and misinformation about sexuality and sexual behavior abound, and staff members are not immune to this. A good staff training program should include a review of basic anatomy and physiology, information on sexual behavior, psychosexual development, sexual problems, and sexual orientations and variations, all in an atmosphere that promotes a certain comfort level. Desensitizing experiences can be a part of the training. Attendance at an SAR (Sexual Attitude Restructuring) Workshop or a similar workshop that uses tapes, films, and discussion is one means of providing this experience. Often, persons who feel that they are open-minded about sexuality realize through the desensitization experience that there are areas of sexuality and sexual behavior that elicit negative feelings in them. The goal of desensitization is to help individuals become aware of where their own lines of acceptance are drawn and how this might affect their acceptance of others' behaviors. The choice of changing their own behavior is up to them, but it is hoped that their acceptance of others' behaviors would be expanded.

The training sessions should also encourage the participants to examine their own values, beliefs, and feelings, with the goal of self-awareness and self-knowledge. An added benefit might be that of increasing the individual's own comfort and tolerance levels. It is imperative that staff persons working with disturbed adolescents be comfortable with themselves as persons, as sexual beings, and as individuals with their own unique tolerances and intolerances. Adolescents are very sensitive to discrepancies between what is felt and what is said.

The staff already has a knowledge of adolescent development and the idiosyncrasies of adolescents. An important part of staff training is to review this knowledge in relation to the development of a sexual identity. It is important during these sessions to relate the physiological and hormonal changes during this stage with the insecurities that adolescents often feel about their bodies. The general insecurity prevalent during this time is heightened in regard to sex and sexuality, and the training should prepare staff persons to minimize this as much as possible in the disturbed adolescent.

Another area that should be explored during the training sessions is the fears and apprehensions of the staff that encouraging adolescents to explore their sexuality is encouraging uncontrolled sexual behavior. Some staff persons might feel that because the residents now have information they will act out sexually. The goal of a human sexuality program with disturbed adolescents is to encourage the development of their sexual identities. Some might abuse the information and knowledge, but this does not justify withholding it from them. It is also helpful to remind staff that adolescents often enjoy shocking adults and that adult reaction usually begets more shocks. Staff should be prepared for extensive testing behavior early in a human sexuality program.

Ideally, an outgrowth of staff training is a commitment on the part of staff persons to a human sexuality program for the residents. Without this commitment, the program cannot be implemented in a truly meaningful way. In addition to this commitment, there needs to be administrative resolve and support. The leadership of the administration is a crucial factor in program development and implementation. Administrators are able to implement policies that can facilitate the establishment of meaningful programs. They must provide the time and the coverage necessary for staff training.

ROLE OF ADMINISTRATION

Beyond the immediate training and program support, the administration needs to be involved in creating the total milieu. A supportive administration will change the policies he/she is able to change and will creatively work around those which cannot be changed. In addition, an administration can provide leadership in efforts to change those institutional policies which are no longer functional or which impede the maintenance of a therapeutic environment. Specifically, administrative action is necessary to help provide the residents with appropriate social interaction, both within and outside of the institution. Also, the physical layout of most institutions is not conducive to privacy. That there are institutional reasons for this does not negate the importance of privacy to adolescents and to their developing sexual identities. Without administrative support, it is difficult, if not impossible, to create a milieu conducive to a good human sexuality program.

PROGRAMS FOR RESIDENTS

Once the administration and staff are committed and properly prepared, the next step is to begin a program for the residents. This should include specific knowledge, feelings, relationships, values clarification, and honest and open discussion of all matters that seem appropriate as indicated by the interests of the group and the expertise of the leader. The most important aspect of this program is that it is an *affirmation* of human sexuality. Specifics such as areas to be covered, how long the sessions should last, who should lead the groups, and who should be in the groups will be very much dictated by the institution itself — its size, its age range, its resources, etc. There are, however, some areas of caution and advice worth mentioning. The ideal situation calls for small mixed groups of residents of about the same developmental level. Generally, younger adolescents will be less interested in details. It is often disrupting to include too great a range of ages. In essence, it is very important to pay careful attention to the group composition and the group dynamics.

It is a mistake to plan the residents' program as a one-time effort. It must be ongoing and someone must be available at all times. This suggests that staff persons act as leaders of the group sessions, although there are reasons to suggest that outside persons might be more effective in generating open discussion. Perhaps a team approach of a staff person and an outside person would be a good option. Regardless of the format, the leader's openness, honesty, and comfort in dealing with sexuality will be most crucial in facilitating the same qualities in the group. The effect and the benefit of this will be enhanced if a male and a female act as co-leaders. This often helps the comfort level of the male and female adolescents and can set good role models.

Flexibility is a great virtue in a group leader. It is more important to answer all the questions and to speak to all the concerns of the adolescents than to cover a specified amount of material. The authors have found that they have been able to cover all the necessary material by incorporating much of it into answers to questions that inevitably come up. An open-ended contract with the group to schedule wanted and/or needed additional sessions is one way to build in insurance that the material can be covered. Another helpful source of information for the adolescents is resource materials, which should be available at all times. Books are useful as a means of answering some questions and raising others, and their open presence and their availability serve to remind staff and residents alike that exploring one's sexual identity in this environment is accepted and encouraged.

RESPONDING TO SEXUAL BEHAVIORS

After preparing staff persons and instituting a program for residents — both with administrative support — there will still be areas that will be controversial, as is the case in human sexuality programs in other settings. The issues of masturbation, homosexuality, heterosexuality, and sexual acting out are the most difficult on which to get agreement. Masturbation, perhaps the most common means of sexual expression in adolescents, is often discouraged on moral and religious grounds. Another common reason for discouragement is that it is solitary sex and therefore works against the adolescent learning to relate to others. The authors concur with Diane Brashear that masturbation is good and that it "can be important, helpful, comforting and good training to prepare an individual for later, more involved sexual, other-directed responses."[5] Staff persons should feel free to allow disturbed adolescents to masturbate if they so desire. Self-affirmation can be one of the positive results of masturbation, and disturbed adolescents certainly need to have their selves affirmed.

Some adolescents, in experimenting with their new sexual urges, have experiences with members of the same sex. This often causes concern because the adolescent is not able to put it in perspective (nor is he/she usually able to get any adult help in this regard). The result is fear and guilt that the adolescent is a homosexual. While same-sex relationships are created in part by institutional policy, they are happening in response to some need. The behavior will not be changed by disapproving or outlawing it. Same-sex behavior should not be handled in a sensational manner. The behavior is often situational homosexuality and will disappear when other sexual options are made available. For example, in institutions for adolescent girls from multiproblem families where there was no consistent relationship with a parent figure, residents often form their own families within the institution. Father roles are given to the butch girls and mother roles are given to the femmes. The breakdown is more fluid with children's roles. In such situations, there is sexual activity between parents and across families. The bonds are surprisingly strong. Despite this, when the girls leave the institution, most return to their former heterosexual interests.

It is important for staff persons to examine their own attitudes toward same-sex behavior and how these attitudes affect their work with adolescents. An adolescent needs to feel free from adult judgment before being able to approach an adult on this matter. The availability and openness of staff persons to discuss same-sex behavior are important in helping the adolescent sort out responses to sexual overtures and prepare for the possible forced encounter. The openness of staff toward same-sex behavior is especially important with disturbed adolescents who are already experiencing unusual difficulty in their emotions and relationships.

The same, of course, must be said of male-female behavior and relationships. The role of staff persons is not to discourage or outlaw sexual relationships (and here the distinction between sexual relationships and sex behavior must be noted) but to help these develop appropriately. If appropriate development includes sex between adolescents, then this should be allowed. What is appropriate or therapeutic will be determined by the adolescents involved with the counsel of staff persons.

Some institutionalized adolescents seek attention through inappropriate sexual behavior. They are often overtly sexual with staff persons in language and/or actions. Sometimes the specific action is appropriate in itself, but it is when or how the action takes place that makes it inappropriate. One of the residents in an institution for emotionally disturbed adolescent girls, in which one of the authors worked, enjoyed touching staff persons. While that sounds harmless enough, she carried it to extremes by literally hanging on to staff persons, patting them on their buttocks, or managing to nudge their breasts. Each staff person set his/her own personal touching limits with this resident while going out of his/her way to reach out to her in appropriate physical ways. Other examples of this include the residents who fall in love and use their romance to gain prestige with the other adolescents, and the individual who constantly talks about his/her sexual exploits. One may ignore these inappropriate behaviors and reward other behaviors. In the first example, appropriate limits were set, and the staff tried to model appropriate physical contact for the resident.

That emotionally disturbed adolescents are sexual beings cannot be denied even though that fact is ignored in most of the institutions designed to treat them. The paucity of literature in this crucial area is proof enough that sexuality is considered a *healthy* endeavor, i.e. something that can be incorporated once the disturbed adolescent is healthy, rather than a *healthful* endeavor, i.e. something that should be incorporated into the whole treatment environment. This chapter suggests specific steps for incorporating human sexuality into the treatment milieu. There are, of course, difficulties in applying every suggestion to every situation, but do encourage staff persons and administrators to begin to explore ways to help disturbed adolescents integrate their sexuality into their troubled but developing personhoods.

REFERENCES

1. Chapman, A. H. *Management of Emotional Problems of Children and Adolescents*. Philadelphia: J. B. Lippincott Co., 1974, p. 10.
2. Holmes, Donald J. *The Adolescent in Psychotherapy*. Boston: Little, Brown & Co., 1964.
3. *Ibid.*, p. 30.
4. Lambert, B. Geraldine, Rothschild, Barbara, Altlant, Richard and Green, Laurence B. *Adolescence*. Montery, Calif.: Brooks/Cole Publishing Co., 1972.
5. Brashear, Diane B. "Honk! If you masturbate!", *Siecus Report*, 3(2), pp. 13-14, November, 1974.

Chapter Sixteen

MENTALLY HANDICAPPED

WINIFRED KEMPTON AND LINDA CARELLI

IT is very difficult today to present a generalized account of adolescents in institutions for the mentally retarded; to be specific about their sexuality is even more difficult. Thirty years ago, when their care was mainly custodial, a description would have been more simple. In those days the mentally retarded individual was traditionally committed to an institution for any of several reasons:

1. when the family was unable to cope with its retarded member;
2. when there was no one to care for him/her adequately;
3. when it was believed he/she would receive better training and be "better off with his own kind"; or
4. when it was necessary to protect him/her from getting into trouble — a man from committing crimes of assault and sex, a woman from having a baby. (One of the present authors remembers those days with guilt when she helped commit mentally retarded girls to a Pennsylvania institution for "child-bearing women.")

Today, reasons for institutionalization are being seriously examined, and the scene is changing. New methods of helping the mentally retarded and their families are being introduced almost everywhere. However, institutions vary widely in their rate of transition; no two are similiar enough to warrant accurate conclusions on our mentally retarded adolescent population. Some insights can be gleaned, however, from observations made during consultative visits to many institutions for the mentally retarded in the United States and in feedback from institutional staffs during training courses on sexuality.

The Impact of the Normalization Principle

A combination of knowledge (epidemiological and of treatment models), humanitarian views, consumer advocacy, and judicial efforts has made a tremendous impact on society's consciousness of the mentally retarded. Services and care are greatly influenced by the Normalization Principle, i.e. using methods as culturally normal as possible to establish and/or maintain appropriate personal behaviors and characteristics. It implies both a process and a goal in an attempt to develop behavior and appearance that come as close to being normal as circumstances and the person's behavioral potential permit. The principle also includes human management to elicit such behavior and to reflect techniques enhancing the normalization process (Wolfensberger, 1972).

Normalization at work is demonstrated by the current national policy known as deinstitutionalization. This means —

- preventing both unnecessary admission to and retention in institutions;
- finding and developing appropriate alternatives in the community for housing, treatment, training, education, and rehabilitation of the mentally retarded who do not need to be in institutions;
- improving conditions, care, and treatment for those who do need institutional care.

This approach is based on the principle that mentally handicapped persons are entitled to live in the least restrictive environment possible and to lead their lives as normally and independently as possible (General Accounting Office, 1977).

This policy is reflected in legislation in the field of rehabilitation and developmental disabilities since 1963, in the 1975 Title XX Amendment to the Social Security Act, and in the most recent legislation, the Rehabilitation Comprehensive Service and Developmental Disabilities Amendment of 1978.

In spite of these efforts for deinstitutionalization, many of the mentally retarded continue to live in such places. A few of the many roadblocks to community living are community attitudes, lack of client readiness programs, and insufficient funding. The progress of deinstitutionalization is uncertain. Moreover the impact on society's consciousness noted earlier has affected the services and care for the mentally retarded still in institutions. For example, in many places each resident must now have an individualized habilitation plan. Also, many managers are trying to make the institutional environment as normal as possible.

A 1975 study found that approximately 168,300 mentally retarded individuals live in public institutions (General Accounting Office Report, 1977). The largest number of deinstitutionalized individuals are borderline and mildly mentally retarded; the institutionalized are the more severely and profoundly mentally retarded. Though this figure is not broken down by age, adolescents form a large group.

The Mentally Retarded Adolescent

To understand the sexual adolescent who is mentally retarded we should first consider a definition of mental retardation as given by the American Association on Mental Deficiency: "significantly sub-average, general intellectual functioning existing concurrently with deficits in adaptative behavior and manifested during the developmental period" (National Association of Retarded Citizens, 1973). The descriptive terminology varies, but it should mainly be regarded as a convenience in communication and should be handled cautiously (Gallagher, 1976). The term *Educable Mentally Retarded* (EMR) is sometimes used to designate the mentally handicapped person who has apparent potential to learn to care for him/herself and to gain some degree of self-sufficiency, possibly to learn to read and write; the term *Trainable Mentally Retarded* (TMR) implies less basic abilities for academic learning and adaptability. *Mildly* and *Moderately Retarded* (IQ less than 50) as opposed to *Severely* and *Profoundly Retarded* are terms commonly used today as slightly refined descriptions, but they are not taken very seriously by people working with the retarded. Experience has shown that the level of adaptive and intellectual abilities cannot be measured consistently, since they vary greatly both within the individual and in comparison with others. The expression *a person who is retarded* is becoming more desirable than *the retarded* because it asserts that these are people with a handicap rather than an all-encompassing characteristic that places them outside all bounds of normalcy.

While mentally retarded adolescents are generally less adaptive and have less intellectual ability than their nonretarded counterparts, there is no difference in their basic sex drive. They are born with the same natural sexual desires. Therefore, mentally retarded adolescents have sexual feelings, are exposed to sexual messages and experiences, and are, indeed, sexual people. Also, like the rest of the population, they may or may not have a strong interest in sex; they may go through life without strong orgiastic experiences (Johnson, 1973).

However, the sexual behavior of retarded adolescents differs from their nonhandicapped peers in several ways. First is the pattern of development in their adolescent years. Murry Morgenstern makes the following statement in "The Psychosexual Development of the Retarded":

> Within broad limits, the retardate's development follows the same schedule as the normal person's, except that the retarded person requires more time to advance from one stage to another and, because of his deficits and smaller store of capacities, has less tolerance for stress, more readily accessible masses of anxiety, weaker ego strength, and poorer relationships to people and objects. The retarded person may never be as completely attuned to people, as the normal person, but *this may be as much the result of his living experiences and overall deficits, as of developmental omissions.* On the physical level, interference with the retardate's growth and development is attributable to chromosome anomalies, inborn errors of metabolism, genetic aberrations, cortical insults, and the like. On the psychological level, interference with development is attributable to insufficient ego, indifference to environment, environmental deprivation, inability to shift thinking, and lack of discrimination of self. (Morgenstern, 1973)

Therefore, retarded children usually reach adolescence far less prepared for its stresses than so-called normal youths, and certainly ill-prepared for coping with emotional and social involvements. The needs to develop social sexual identity, to strengthen their existing sense of identity, to assume a sex role, and to achieve a measure of independence exist for the retarded as well. These goals, however, cannot be achieved quickly or easily, and some people may never achieve them.

Dependence upon parents or caretakers remains almost total as retarded children grow into adolescence, preventing them from developing into sexually mature adults. They are rejected because of their handicaps, overprotected, and segregated by sex sometimes because of anxieties roused by the manifestations of their sexuality. Consequently, they are deprived of the opportunities for social learning that their peers use to develop social skills and self-confidence. The results are that many retarded adolescents are childlike in their dependence on others, nondiscriminatory in forming relationships, and generally lacking in social skills.

To identify a pattern of sexual behavior for the retarded adolescent, as Erikson does for the normal (Erikson, 1950), is virtually impossible. We do not know what the social-sexual potential is for retarded individuals because of the limitations traditionally placed on them. Their basic learning abilities vary from none at all to the borderline person who can hardly be identified as retarded — a gamut that defies a generalized description. Nevertheless, some simple assumptions about the sexual adaptation of retarded adolescents can be made.

We have observed that most severely retarded people (about 10 to 15% of the retarded population) can be taught at best only basic sexually related activities, such as proper hygiene, proper techniques, places for masturbation, and socially acceptable methods of physical contact with others. The spontaneous sexual activities of profoundly retarded persons are necessarily almost entirely confined to autoeroticism. Most of them enjoy touching and cuddling. It is unlikely that they can ever participate in organized social activities involving easy communication or closeness with a group or an individual. Sexual encounters between severely retarded persons are haphazard and disorganized (Jaffe, 1976).

On the other hand, the mildly retarded and many of those moderately so are capable of socializing, dating, marrying, and having children, although parenting presents far greater obstacles to them than to the general population (Floor et al., 1975).

According to "Sex and the Mentally Handicapped" in *Physicians World, October, 1974,* experts believe that 15 percent of the higher level retarded population can understand sex education principles (Brenton, 1974). Yet, retarded adolescents reach adulthood in almost total ignorance of sexual matters. Dozens of cases have been reported in which a retarded couple marries not knowing the act of sexual intercourse exists.

Lack of Acceptance of the Mentally Retarded Adolescent's Sexuality

While much progress has been made in habilitative services in general, this has not reached sexuality. Often, integration of sexuality with adaptive and psychosocial development does not exist. The institutionalized mentally retarded adolescent is barred from achieving sexual identity and developing social relationships.

The authors' experiences in institutions for the mentally retarded provide many illustrations of the repression of sexuality and sexual adjustment in the adolescent. Such illustrations cover habilitative planning and program implementation, both on a daily basis in the institution and as preparation (or lack of) for community living. The overall pervasive attitude toward any expression by an individual in an institution is governed by the concern that the expression not cause disruption or create a behavior problem. Thus the adolescent who demonstrates sexual curiosity, anxieties, or fears is watched cautiously lest a problem develop.

In fairness it should be stated that such attitudes are reinforced by working conditions in institutions with low staff/client ratios or those not reflective of client needs. Also, while there may be direct-care staff and professional staff supportive of sexual awareness as healthy development for the mentally retarded adolescent in one setting of the institution, in another it may be discouraged, i.e. dorm setting vs. social setting.

The individual attitudes of the staff often vary widely within an institution, as shown in one study of the attitudes of direct-care staff and of academicians toward sexual behavior. The direct-care staff tended to be conservative and the academics more liberal toward sex education for the mentally retarded. In fact, the authors of this study report that "a large percentage of staff members feel that no sexual behavior on the part of residents is acceptable" (Mitchell et al., 1978).

Attention must be given to staff training, which again varies widely. In some of the smaller, more progressive institutions, many of the staff have been exposed to some training programs on the sexuality of their residents. In others a few selected staff are given training, then assigned some responsibility for setting up in-service and education programs for the residents. Some institutions almost completely ignored the subject. As implied by the study of staff attitudes noted above, training will require an assessment of staff attitudes, and then the training program must address these attitudes.

Institutional Policies on Sexual Behavior

Because the mental retardation field is in a period of change, policies on handling the sexual behavior of the residents vary widely among institutions. Many have no policies; many are weighing the need for them; some have formed committees and written guidelines for their staffs.

The authors have observed that all institutional staffs flounder in one aspect of behavior or another, whether there are established policies or not. As long as individual differences in attitudes exist, it is nearly impossible to expect total consistency within any staff. However, establishing policies represents some recognition of the sexual aspects of institutional life for the mentally retarded. Improvement is seen in many institutions, and the number of staff involved is growing.

Sexual Behaviors in the Institutional Setting

In spite of the many differences, some problems involving the sexuality of the mentally retarded adolescent are common to all institutions. Three specific areas of sexual behavior engaged in by residents arouse the concern of staff members:

1. masturbatory habits
2. heterosexual behavior/relationships
3. homosexual behavior/relationships

Masturbation. Masturbation as a means of expressing sexual desire is becoming more acceptable in many institutions. At least, the kind of harsh punishment dealt out twenty years ago (such as using boxing gloves to prevent masturbation) no longer exists, to our knowledge. However, problems still do. First, attitudes of a staff may vary from sharply reprimanding, to ignoring completely (even if inappropriate), to teasing, to an understanding tolerance. This inconsistency may confuse adolescents and cause guilt feelings. Second, a complaint often heard from staff is "So we *have* assumed a policy to accept masturbation as long as it is private — but where can our residents find privacy?" In normalizing the institutional setting, home-like furnishings have been added; in some institutions large bedrooms or dormitories have been converted (in some cases partitioned) to make six to eight individual rooms; more normalized clothing has been supplied. Bathrooms vary — some have doors on the toilet and shower areas; others continue to have none. In spite of these changes, lack of privacy remains a major roadblock to allowing individual masturbating activity.

Other problems involve the inability of some adolescents to learn to masturbate in private, especially those who are profoundly retarded and are unable to learn other modes of behavior. Some of them cannot reach a climax. Some girls injure themselves by inserting sharp objects in their vaginas not understanding effective ways of stimulating their clitorises. Should the adolescents be taught how to masturbate? This can be an explosive issue for institutional staff.

Heterosexual Behavior/Relationships. Adolescent heterosexual relationships are still regarded anxiously by many institutional staffs, although many retarded girls and boys do not have the social skills to become intimately involved with each other. As noted above, they need to learn simple techniques for communicating with each other and having fun together. Sexual intercourse leading to babies is hardly their goal of social relationship at this stage of their social development. However, learning to handle their strong sexual urges should be an important aspect of their training, as well as developing the social skills they so sadly lack. Some institutions are making attempts to provide this help, but there are too few of them.

For example, dances were held on a weekly basis at one institution. These could have been primary social events providing training situations for developing appropriate social relationships. Instead, a male adolescent would inappropriately hug the author, often following this by grabbing and pushing. Sometimes their physical closeness, even in a fast dance, expressed strong sexual feelings. The author soon learned that an informal policy existed discouraging staff from dancing with the residents. Thus, while the institution could have built a favorable emotional environment and a healthy model, it actually neglected opportunities to teach appropriate interpersonal relationships to residents. The mentally retarded adolescents in this setting were searching for recognition, acceptance, and affection and could have learned through perceptive direction and development of models.

In this same institution, progress in allowing the sexes to spend some time together seemed to occur when a coed cottage was arranged. On closer examination, it was learned that male adolescents were moved into a building with women, primarily adult, some elderly. Asking one of the males after the move how he liked living with women elicited the comment "Don't like these old women" — a very appropriate response. Again, a situation that could have been a positive one for the development of appropriate social relationships, an important aspect of adolescence, was hampered.

Homosexual Behavior/Relationships. Traditionally, homosexual behavior is a common phenomenon in all sexually segregated institutions, and those for the mentally retarded are no exception. In general, staff are more repressive of heterosexual than homosexual behavior, for the latter won't produce unwanted babies. Some staff may punish simple acts of heterosexual behavior that adolescents outside institutions indulge in freely, then ignore homosexual activity frowned on by the community. This can be confusing to the mentally retarded. Staff who are understanding and relaxed about sexual behavior still face problems involving homosexual activities. However, how much of this sexual behavior is based on early conditioning, lack of social skills, and few opportunities to be with the other sex? Would the adolescent really prefer homosexuality in any setting? What about the same-sexed couple who show strong sexual feelings for each other? How far should they be permitted to go? Should staff interfere when an aggressive adolescent seems to be taking over a passive partner who apparently is not suffering from the relationship?

Sterilization of the Adolescent in Institutions

It has been common practice for institutions to perform hysterectomies or tubal ligations on mentally retarded girls and vasectomies on boys soon after they reach adolescence. Anxiety that they may become parents has been so great that the practice has been indiscriminate. New policies are being established, and today few sterilizations are being performed in institutional settings. Some hysterectomies are being performed on profoundly mentally retarded girls as a medical procedure to prevent their experiencing some of the troublesome side effects of menstruation. The condition of some emotionally disturbed retarded girls is aggravated during the menstrual period, causing great difficulty for themselves and those near them. There is something to be said also about the rights of the caretakers who have to clean the bloodstains of a profoundly mentally retarded girl who not only cannot care for herself but who uses the menstrual period in such an extreme manner. These hysterectomies are not considered a means of preventing pregnancy but a medical procedure to improve the girl's condition.

Birth Control

Birth control probably is not an issue for the adolescent girl who is severely mentally retarded. It should only be considered if there is clear indication that the individual is or will be sexually active through intercourse. Because such a girl is continuously supervised in the institution and because her interest in sex is primarily autoerotic, intercourse is unlikely to occur.

Sexual Knowledge

Research done by Hall and Morris demonstrates that mentally retarded adolescents in institutions have considerably less social-sexual knowledge than those living at home. Such knowledge appears to decrease as they stay longer in the institution. However, this research indicates a higher score for mentally retarded adolescents living in coed facilities in institutions than those in same-sex housing (Hall and Morris, 1976).

Conclusion

This chapter points out some important considerations involved with the sexuality of the mentally retarded, institutionalized adolescent. To demonstrate these points, here is an outline of a typical day for these individuals. Schedules vary among large institutions, but they usually follow this general pattern, which provides insight into the recognition of and attention to sexuality:

Early am 7-8:00 am	• Waken in a dorm room of 20-30 individuals of the same sex, or (in some places) 4-8 individuals in a large room divided by partitions.
Breakfast	• Breakfast in same cottage/building (same sex) or in a dining area in another building, which may be coed, but individuals are usually required to sit with the same-sex group from their own cottage.
Program	• School, prevocational, or daily living classes; most are within the institution; a few residents ride buses to outside programs. Those who do go out are often segregated by sex on either side of the bus though this may not be the case in a public school or other agency-sponsored bus. Coed situations usually exist in the program settings.
	• However, if the program is in the institution, the adolescents may return to their cottages/buildings for lunch and thus again be segregated by sex.
Dinner	• May be in the cottages, thus probably segregated by sexes, or coed in a dining area of another building.
Recreation	• Often organized in the evening in the cottage/buildings, thus primarily segregated by sex. Other activities, such as dances, are planned in a central recreation facility such as a gym and are often coed.
Other Social/ Leisure Time Activities	• TV in the dorms (or residences), again segregated. Boy Scouts, Girl Scouts — again segregated. Trips (to movies, plays, ballgames) are usually segregated by cottages or buildings especially in transportation to and from the activity, but not always.
Bath, Snack, Bed	• Again, segregated by dorm or cottage.

A day's activities may include individual therapies and services, i.e. physical therapy, social work services. Weekends may include church for some residents, social activities, visits from families, and recreation.

Sex education programs do exist in some institutions, often integrated in Daily Care of Skills Training Programs with emphasis on body parts, sex roles, hygiene, and appropriate settings for masturbation. These programs may meet in weekly one-hour sessions for six weeks or more, but only selected individuals may attend.

The adolescent's need to develop sexual identity and appropriate interpersonal relationships is hardly met in the above situations. Coed programs and social activities provide too few opportunities to socialize with the other sex, and there is little opportunity to develop sexual identity and appropriate relationships.

An attempt has been made in this chapter to present a generalized status of the attitude toward sexuality in the institution setting. While further exploration and studies are needed to expand the scope presented, it appears obvious that normalization in sexuality and/or sexual behaviors continues to encounter strains and barriers.

REFERENCES

Brenton, M. Sex and the mentally handicapped. *Physicians World*, 1974.

Erikson, E. H. *Childhood in Society*. New York: Norton, 1950.

Floor, L., Baxter, D., Rosen, M., & Zisfein. A survery of marriages among previously institutionalized retardates. *Mental Retardation*, 1975, 13.

Gallagher, J. J. The sacred and profane use of labeling. *Mental Retardation*, 1976, 14.

General Accounting Office of the United States, *Returning the Mentally Disabled to the Community: Government Needs to do More*, HRD-76-152, January, 1977.

Hall, Judy and Morris, Helen. Sexual knowledge and attitudes of institutionalized and noninstitutionalized retarded adolescents, *American Journal of Mental Deficiency*, Vol. 80, No. 1, 1976.

Jaffe, D. Unpublished paper. Includes quotation from THE RIGHT TO LOVE, a report from England., 1975.

Johnson, W. Sex education of the mentally retarded. In de la Cruz and La Veck (Eds.), *Human Sexuality and the Mentally Retarded*. New York: Brunner/Mazel, 1973.

Kempton, W. and Morgenstern, Murry. The psychosexual development of the retarded. In de la Cruz and La Veck (Eds.), *Human Sexuality and the Mentally Retarded.* New York: Brunner/Mazel, 1973.

Mitchel, L., Doctor, R. M. & Butler, D. C. Attitudes of caretakers toward the sexual behavior of mentally retarded persons. *American Journal of Mental Deficiency,* 1978, Vol. 83, No. 3.

Mulhern, Thomas. Survey of reported sexual behavior and policies characterizing residential facilities for retarded citizens. *American Journal of Mental Deficiency,* Vol. 79 No. 6, 1975.

National Association of Retarded Citizens. *Facts on Mental Retardation,* Arlington, Texas: National Association of Retarded Citizens, n.d.

Wolfensberger, Wolf. *The Principle of Normalization in Human Services.* Toronto, Canada: National Institute of Mental Retardation, 1972.

BIBLIOGRAPHY

Kempton, Winifred. *A Teachers Guide to Sex Education for Persons with Learning Disabilities,* North Scituate, Massachusetts: Duxbury Press, 1975.

Rehabilitation, Comprehensive Services & Developmental Disabilities Amendments of 1978, Public Law 95-602, HR-12467, No. 6, 1978.

Title XX Amendments (Social Services) to the Social Security Act, 1975.

Chapter Seventeen

CHRONICALLY ILL AND DISABLED

Larry Lister

MANY issues must be taken into consideration when attempting to understand the sexuality of chronically ill or disabled adolescents and young adults who are in institutions. As a point of reference for the remarks to follow, consider the case of John, a seventeen year old tuberculosis patient who had been admitted to a TB hospital following his collapse at the end of a 20-mile hike. In spite of his robust outward appearance, John had an advanced condition that required months of hospitalization.

In his initial assessment at the time of admission, the social worker learned that John had recently arrived in Hawaii from his home on one of the Pacific islands. He was living with an aunt and uncle while he attended school. John impressed the social worker as a shy and pleasant youth who had something of a problem with the English language, but this was easily overcome with repetitions of some words. John was assigned a tutor to continue with his school work, his local relatives were concerned and in contact, and as he gained strength following his weak condition at the time of admission, it appeared that John's hospital stay would be long but — with adequate planning for his psychosocial needs — unremarkable.

However, the social worker was contacted one morning by the head nurse, who reported a rather bizarre episode that had occurred the previous night. Apparently in an impulsive manner, John had leaped on the bed of an elderly patient and had grabbed him by the scrotum. The staff were concerned on several counts, both as to the reasons for John's highly inappropriate behavior and also because the elderly victim had, in addition to TB, a serious heart condition. Needless to say, the whole episode had caused a considerable stir on the ward the previous night.

After receiving the nurse's call, the social worker went to the ward and found John doing his artwork at his bedside. The ward was settled and life was proceeding as usual, so the social worker invited John to join him in his office for a talk about the events of the night before. Once in the office, the social worker informed John of his understanding of the episode, and John shyly and noddingly confirmed the report as accurate. In the discussion that ensued — which, as in other previous talks with John, was mainly one sided, with the social worker eliciting nods, brief remarks, and a puzzled look if John didn't understand — the social worker became convinced that John's behavior was not an expression of erotic interest in the elderly patient but was an act of aggression of a still quite psychosexually immature boy. This assessment was supported by other information the social worker had available from the admission study and subsequent observations of John's behavior by other staff.

Active intervention was called for, both to assure that there would be no repeat of the attack on the elderly patient and to prevent John from being stigmatized by other patients or even by staff as in some was a deviant. The male social worker explicitly discussed with John that there could not be a repeat of the episode of the night before. He explained that the older patient had a heart problem and that it could be a shock to him to have his scrotum suddenly grabbed. The puzzled look on John's face led the social worker to clarify that John could not grab the other patient's balls (the puzzled look was replaced by a look of comprehension), but the social worker went on to explain that as far as the hospital was concerned, John could handle his own balls and do whatever he wished with his own body. The social worker continued to explain that the hospital understood that young men could feel cooped up being in a hospital for a long time and that it was quite natural for them to masturbate (further clarified as beating off, which John understood). The social worker then went on to extract a promise from John that there would not be repeat attacks on any other patients in the future.

This part of the interview thus sufficiently resolved, they continued to discuss other issues of importance. Earlier planning for John had provided him with the tutor to continue his school work, the hospital had made a guitar available when he had indicated an interest, and some art supplies had been accumulated, since he was able to occupy many hours in painting and drawing, an activity for which he demonstrated considerable talent. However, it was determined that John had few art supplies and no money of his own with which to purchase equipment. It was also apparent that John's physical energy had returned to his more usual level but that his activities in the hospital were mainly sedentary.

As the social worker explored some of these issues, he learned of the limited supply of art materials and an additional piece of information when John revealed that his mother, who still lived on the home island, believed his TB had been caused by his playing football. She was consequently sending the message to the local relatives that John must not play football in the future.

As a result of this information, the social worker — in conjunction with the tutor and the occupational therapist — devised a means of securing a steady supply of art materials, with the tutor and occupational therapist initiating plans for a show of John's art in the hospital lobby. Concurrently, the social worker consulted John's physician and arranged for him to talk with local relatives and to write a letter to John's mother, reassuring her that the TB had not been caused by playing football and that, in fact, once John was well, it would be good for him to be further involved in football and in other sports of his interest. With the resultant approval of the relatives, a football was made available to John for his use on the hospital grounds while he remained an inpatient.

The outcome of the multiple efforts in John's case was positive. There was no repetition of the impulsive behavior with the elderly patient or any other patients. John was not stigmatized or rejected by his ward peers and, in fact, could be found playing cards, guitar, or football with groups of patients at various times. His art show was a success, attended by staff, other patients, and several of John's relatives. John was discharged after several more months of in-hospital care and, as an outpatient, he dropped by the social worker's office on return visits to the clinic to let it be known that he was doing all right and, in fact, was on his high school football team.

John's case serves to illustrate a number of points. It is important to recognize that the "chronically ill child spends most of his life in the community."[1] Few chronically ill* young people are reared in institutions, although, since by definition a chronic condition is "marked by long duration or frequent recurrence,"[2] there may be significant episodes of institutional care for many chronically ill youths. It must be recognized that the terms *chronic illness* and *disability* refer to a wide range of health conditions. In John's case, for example, what is termed a chronic illness was manifested by an acute onset in adolescence and, other than for routine follow-up, would be expected to have minimal impact on his future ability to function. John's TB is thus a remarkably different condition from that of a cerebral palsy or muscular dystrophy patient, whose entire life experience prior to adolescence will have been affected by the special care and attention required as a result of the limitations imposed by the illness. Different, too, will be the past experiences and future prospects of patients such as the spinal cord injured, who, from the time of injury, must face the future with a permanent paralysis. Each of these groups of patients, then, must be considered with regard to how their sexuality has been affected throughout the entire life cycle, at and beyond a certain traumatic point in time, at any time of institutional residence, and prospectively into their individual futures.

What is meant by the all-encompassing term *sexuality* must also be clarified. At least four important "spheres" of sexuality can be delineated: (1) the biological and reproductive; (2) the spheres of gender identity and sex role behavior; (3) the sphere of the influence of the sex drive, including the erotic and sensual aspects of sexuality; and (4) sexual activities.

---

*In this chapter, chronic illness and disability refer to physical problems, rather than to emotional, behavioral, or intellectual problems, though with due recognition to their interrelationship.

The Biological and Reproductive Sphere

In the social work intervention activity with John, little attention was given to the biological and reproductive sphere. John was a postpubescent adolescent, who would clearly be capable of reproducing and functioning physically in the future. The same could not be said of many other chronically ill adolescents, so health team professionals may need to give much greater attention in this sphere of sexuality when adolescents and young adults are institutionalized. There are a number of chronic conditions that prevent or limit the ability to reproduce. For example, there is a high risk of impotence due to disease of the peripheral blood vessels in diabetic males which, for the adolescent or young adult, has crucial implications for his future life.[3] Since diabetes is an inherited disease, even in cases where reproduction is possible, the fear of producing a diabetic offspring may well impose a handicapping anxiety about intercourse on the part of any diabetic male or female.

Another example of an impediment to reproduction is that encountered by many spinal cord injury victims.[4] While pregnancy is usually possible, complications in giving birth and in raising a child can easily interfere with the expectation of anything like the usual sexual activity of the nondisabled. For spinal cord injured males, there is a possibility that no erection can be achieved, combined with a possibility of no sensations of orgasm. Thus, both the prospects of reproduction and/or the anticipation of sensual pleasure may be denied these youths.

Gender Identity and Sex Role Behavior

The sexual spheres of gender identity and sex role behavior are crucial areas for all adolescents and young adults. Consideration for this sphere was well illustrated in the intervention activity in John's case. The social worker was concerned that John not be stigmatized within the hospital in any way that would create for him a deviant self-concept. There were also planned efforts to further maximize his interests and talents in art and music as well as in athletics (realizing the potential that his athletic skill would have for providing him an easy entry back into his high school peer group).

Again, however, consideration must be given to the type of

chronic condition and its impact on the total life of the individual. Long before they ever come to the institution, many chronically ill youths will have had a lifetime of experiences upon which their sexual identity is based. For example, when identity is thought of as the sense of individuality, separateness, and autonomy of the individual, consider how child-rearing patterns have had to interfere with the accomplishment of this sense of a separate selfness in many cerebral palsy youngsters who, according to Carson, are "carried over the shoulder of their parents to the period of preadolescence — in their psychosexual development a post-oedipal development is an exception — so much attention and energy has had to be given to the functions of eating and eliminating that they often remain the chief avenues of sexual gratification even in adulthood. Genital sexuality is often hampered until these adolescents can work through their feelings regarding extended handling of their sexual organs by their parents during ages when there should be a quiescence in parent-child intimacy."[5] The whole issue of autonomy from parents, so crucial to identity formation, can be problematic for youths who have the psychosocial need and yet who are forced by their health condition into prolonged physical dependency.

The peer group, by its reactions to and interactions with the adolescent, also has a profound impact on the identity formation of each group member. Often the chronically ill youth's experiences have been so influenced by the constraints of the physical condition that his or her identity includes a central disabled, or "sick-role," component. Some aspects of this identity will have been repeatedly reinforced through life in special education classes, summer camping programs, episodes of institutional care, and other experiences that highlight the disabled aspect of identity through primary association with children with similar afflictions. Since this can be a limiting world, forcing a too constructed identity, attempts are currently underway nationwide to mainstream these children into the more usual social systems of life. However, it must be remembered how crucial are the reactions of *all* peers in forging the individuals' identity; many chronic conditions have, as noted by Travis, "stigmatizing characteristics, such as the irritating cough and foul flatulence of cystic fibrosis, the loss of hair from radiation for leukemia, the obesity and growth of facial hair from steroids for kidney disease, the smell of urine surrounding the incontinent youth with spina bifida, and the crippling of hemophilia or arthritis or muscular dystrophy — all these create the social situation of the stigmatized."[6]

Many youths will thus enter the institution in various states of identity crisis. It would be safe to say that any inpatient setting serving adolescent patients will be influencing the sexual identity sphere and that principles that were applicable in John's case should be used in work with every adolescent and young adult who requires inpatient care.

Another case example may further illustrate the potential role of the institution in fostering the sexual identity of disabled young people. Bill entered the institution in his early twenties, following an accident that left him permanently paralyzed in the lower half of his body. Prior to his accident, Bill had lived a free lifestyle in a remote area of one of the Hawaiian islands. He had prided himself on his individual self-sufficiency as well as on his ability to "give love" to women. Bill was thus profoundly depressed as he increasingly realized that both his autonomy and his ability to function sexually — the foundations of his identity — were irretrievably lost. The social worker spent long hours with Bill over an extended period of time as the young man vent his feelings and questioned why he should live. Gradually, and partly in response to a concerted team effort in delivering total care, Bill began to be able to discuss other ways in which he could still express love to and receive love from women. Concerted staff efforts had facilitated as many ongoing contacts with his former friends as was possible for Bill, while the social worker, building on Bill's own values, helped him to see where other parts of his body (since he was totally impotent) could not only receive pleasurable sensations but could provide pleasure to the several women who had remained in contact with him. It was not possible for Bill to ever return to the rural surroundings where he had formerly created a home for himself, but the social worker encouraged Bill as he tentatively began to reaccumulate some of his valued possessions to fashion his own environment (reflective of *his* personal identity) within the institution. Gradually Bill's room took on the appearance of the counterculture, with candles, incense, plants, and psychedelic wall hangings creating an atmosphere that was unique within the institution. In this manner, Bill's personal identity was partially maintained and strengthened along with his will to survive and further enhance the other necessary aspects of his newer identity.

The Erotic and Sensual Sphere

As is obvious in the preceding discussion, each sexual sphere overlaps all others. The capacity to reproduce cannot be totally separated from identity or the erotic sphere from the other three spheres identified. Somewhere on their bodies, all chronically ill or disabled adolescent and young adults have the capacity to respond sensuously. All institutional staff providing nursing care to males have encountered the erections — and the frequent concomitant embarrassment — of the young man who is being bathed. These erections may or may not signify erotic arousal (they may be simply reflexive as in cases of spinal cord damage) and rarely do they initiate the response, as occurred in one case, of the nurse who ran gleefully to the physician to report the occurrence of a first postinjury erection in a young quadriplegic patient. Out of context it may appear that the nurse's behavior was inappropriate, yet in the actual situation she was sharing the elation of the patient who had been almost compulsively masturbating for weeks in an attempt to achieve this very goal. It is not uncommon for young quadriplegics to be seductive or — as in the words of one young man, "promiscuous" — during the time their capacity for sexual performance or sensual arousal is in question.

Again, it must be stressed that the institution's role in meeting the sexual needs of chronically ill or disabled persons must be adapted to the total circumstances of the individual. The examples cited have been young men who have already experienced erotic sexuality. The institution's role with younger adolescent patients — or with those patients whose preceding lives have not encouraged sexual development in one or more spheres — must be appropriate to the needs identified. For example, data cited by Wright comparing physically disabled and nondisabled young women, show that a smaller proportion of the disabled had information about sex before age fifteen, fewer were prepared for menstruation, and even fewer had been in love or had dated before age sixteen.[7] These data indicate a lack of information input and a more limited peer-group involvement for the disabled young women, but possibly they also indicate a lower expectation as to the relevance of sexuality to the disabled woman. A case illustrating this point was that of a middle-adolescent girl with cerebral palsy who had spent many years in institutions and who had acquired a belief that she could become pregnant by simply being alone with a man! Not only had this girl come from a family that was fundamentalist in religious orientation, but because of her severe speech problems, she had enjoyed few opportunities for sustained conversations with staff or other patients in the institutions where she had previously lived. As a consequence of this lack of stimulation, she had been labeled as mentally retarded. In the new institution, the female social worker scheduled weekly meetings with the girl to accomplish a number of therapeutic goals. In these discussions, the social worker was able to determine that the girl was at least average in intelligence, that she also had many unanswered questions about various spheres of sexuality. Contrary to assumptions based on the former institution's appraisal of the family background as ultraconservative and sexually repressive, the girl had a healthy curiosity about sex and an intense need to be able to discuss her concerns and her distorted information.

It is highly appropriate for a health care facility to contribute to the sexual health of its patients. Institutions, in reality, vary considerably in the attention they give to the sexual aspects of their patient's lives. Referring again to the initial case vignette of John, it is important to note the social worker's way of handling the episode of John's impulsive attack on the elderly patient. After ascertaining that the attack was not a reflection of any erotic interest on John's part, the social worker went on to discuss with John the hospital's position · with regard to masturbation. What was communicated was that the hospital regarded this as understandable and acceptable behavior for persons who find themselves confined for a period of time. In discussing the issue in this way, the social worker was clearly aware that the boy's religious and cultural background may not have provided any permissiveness to masturbation. Nonetheless, (and without knowing or seeking to know John's own sex practices) the social worker was simply expressing the point of view of the institution, indicating to John that he could make his own decisions about any sexual activity and indicating as well that sex was an issue that could be discussed openly between them.

Sexual Activities

It is important that institutional staff have some discussions and agreements between them as to what they consider permissible sexual activity, the last of the spheres of sexuality that have been identified for this discussion. Because staff are individuals, from various backgrounds and with variations in their own sexual behavior and attitudes, they are not necessarily uniform in what they communicate to patients, nor are they necessarily clear on how they are to respond to the sexual behavior of residents. For example, in a workshop for all levels of staff working in an institution for adolescents (albeit not for chronically ill youths), it was somewhat amazing to the professional staff to hear how punitive were the attitudes of the attendants who had the most frequent and ongoing contact with the resident youths. The attendants were equally surprised at the more liberal — and to them quite unrealistic — attitudes of the professionals. It was clear to the workshop leaders how little communication had occurred among all staff about sexual issues and how necessary it was for them to further clarify their different positions, lest the institutionalized adolescents be caught in the bind of inconsistent messages of what was and was not permissible behavior for them.

Some institutions that serve only adolescent residents have developed written statements for staff, setting forth the policy of the institution with regard to what is and is not permissible and giving guidelines for staff to follow in intervention. In a memo to staff at an institution for children with emotional and behavior problems, it was stated that "sexual language should not be reacted to with shock or surprise, but it should not be accepted by any staff member. Since such language is socially unacceptable, the counselor attempts to help the youngster to substitute some more acceptable form of expression — although the fact of sexuality is not disapproved, it is classified as a private acitivity."[8] While one may disagree with the policy articulated, it nevertheless is spelled out for staff information and, one would hope, debate and ongoing revision. It is true that most institutions caring for chronically ill and disabled youths on a short-term basis would doubtless only be donning a bureaucratic frill to go so far as to write out explicit policies guiding responses to the sexual behavior of their patients. Nonetheless, how do staff respond if a sexual overture is made directly to them? What do staff do if they find two adolescents making love? How do staff handle it if they discover homosexual activity among teenage patients? Not knowing the answers to any of these questions can leave individual staff members taking the path of least resistance, which too often is either repressive action or no action, either of which contributes nothing to the positive sexual development of the patient.

The Institution's Role

Everything that has been said to this point has been intended as a guideline for the role of the institution in understanding and meeting the sexual needs of chronically ill or disabled adolescents and young adults. Indeed, quality, total care to these patients should include an assessment of these youth's need for information about the interrelation of their specific illness with their current and future sexual capacities and limitations. An atmosphere should prevail that facilitates questions and discussion on the part of the patient and where answers and responsive discussions are as thorough about sex-related matters as they are about other aspects of the patient's condition. Such discussions do not automatically occur unless staff are aware of their role in facilitating such dialogues. This point was well illustrated when an experienced staff member reported at a conference an incident in which she was discussing concrete resources with a young renal dialysis patient. There was a pause at the end of their discussion, to which the staff member responded by asking if there was anything else on the patient's mind? He responded simply, "why live?" The worker then asked if he was worried about being impotent, which resulted in a great outpouring of feelings of loss and despair about his future. The worker reported to the conference participants that until she had begun to give more attention to the sexual needs of patients, she would not have felt as free to raise a question such as the one she reported. Patients are keenly aware of what can and cannot be talked about, and many articulate patients have given graphic reports of the avoidance by staff of even blatant attempts by patients to open up discussion on some topic of sexuality.

Even beyond the one-to-one contact of patient and staff, the institution should consider the total environment and how it is structured to facilitate or impede the further sexual development of patients. For example as related to the young person's identity and self-concept, bathing, dressing, and examinations by physicians should be carried out in privacy. The personal appearance of youths should be given consideration by attention to personal grooming and the clothing they are able to wear. Opportunities should not be overlooked to further the development of autonomy, as in the instance of the young man, previously shaved by his parents, who may be taught to shave himself, or the young woman who may spend a profitable hour with a volunteer learning makeup or hair-styling techniques.

The importance of visitors cannot be overlooked. For anyone subjected to long periods of institutional care, the need to retain important links to the community is a vital consideration. With adolescents, where the peer group is so important, and especially for chronically ill youths, where consistency of peer relations can often be fragile, the institution should provide for an atmosphere that is attuned to the needs of this age group. There should be ample provision for privacy, since the confidences of adolescents often must be shared in an atmosphere of great secrecy. Such an atmosphere can be created at a patient's bedside as well as in visiting rooms and lounges.

While providing for necessary privacy, there should also be some communal spaces where hospitalized patients can gravitate to interact with each other and where they may also take visitors, since more frequent visits by peers may be facilitated by providing a variety of stimuli to make their visits appealing, rather than merely obligatory. Such communal meeting places, which can be made inviting through use of wall posters, refrigerators, televisions, games, pool tables, and other appealing furnishings (possibly provided as projects by auxiliaries or community service organizations), can also be of value in encouraging the interaction of some patients who may have few visitors.

Conclusion

Chronically ill youths and young adults experience transitional life crises as do nondisabled persons. A central concern for most adolescents and young adults is certainly their sexuality, in its broadest sense as well as in the more discrete spheres that were discussed in this chapter. Health care staff in institutions have an opportunity both to create environments that are geared to the needs of young persons and to provide individualized attention in each patient's various spheres of sexuality. Total health care, which is directed to the total individual, would still remain partial if not directed toward the recognition and enhancement of that part of the person which is his or her sexuality.

REFERENCES

1. Travis, Georgia. *Chronic Illness in Children, It's Impact on Child and Family*. Stanford, Calif: Stanford University Press, 1976, p. 1.
2. *Webster's New Collegiate Dictionary*. Springfield, Mass: G. & C. Merriam Co., 1977.
3. Kolodny, R. C., C. B. Kahn, H. H. Goldstein & D. M. Barnett. "Sexual Dysfunction in Diabetic Men," *Diabetes*, 23(4) pp. 306-309, April 1974.
4. Singh, S. P. & T. Magner. "Sex and Self: The Spinal Cord Injured." *Rehabilitation Literature*, 36(1), pp. 2-10, January 1975.
5. Carson, Arnold S. "Technical Alterations in the Psychotherapy with an Adolescent Cerebral Palsy Patient," *Mental Hygiene*, XLVIII, pp. 249-256. April 1964.
6. Travis, *op cit.*, p. 62.
7. Wright, Beatrice S. *Physical Disability – A Psychological Approach*. N. Y.: Harper & Row, 1960, p. 90.
8. Lambert, Paul. "Memo to Child Care Workers: Notes on the Management of Sex and Stealing," *Child Welfare*, Vol. LV, No. 5, pp. 329-334. May 1976.

INDEX

A
Abortion, 22-23, 54-55
Administrative concerns, 36-49, 52, 71, 205-206
Adolescent rights, 21, 24, 33
Affection, expression of, 31
Agressive acts, 223-224
Attitudes, sexual (*see* Sexual attitudes)
Attitudes of staff, 17-18, 33-35, 38

B
Birth control, 18-19, 52, 174-175, 219

C
Childhood, discovery of, 7-8
Chronically ill and disabled, 223-225
    biological and reproductive considerations, 227
    errotic factors, 230-232
    gender identity, 227-229
    sexual activities, 232
Contraception, 18-19, 52, 174-175, 219
Correctional facilities, 19, 180-199
    organizational characteristics, 181-186
    problems of residents, 190-199
    resident adaptation, 186-190
    therepeutic intervention, 194-199
Counseling, sexual (*see also* Therepeutic interventions) 104-116
    labeling, 107
    limited information, 114-115
    permission giving, 113-114
    preparation for, 104-105
    suggestion giving, 115-116

D
Deinstitutionalization, 101
Desexualization in institutions
    ethics of, 27-35
    prevention of, 32-35
Disabled (*see* Chronically ill)
Dominance through sex, 192
Door openers in sex education, 61-62

E
Emotionally disturbed, institutions for, 200-209
    administrative concerns, 205-206
    programs for residents, 206-207
    sexual behavior in, 207-209
    sexual repression in, 200-201
    staff training, 203-205
Environment, impersonality of, 30
Ethics of desexualization, 27-35
Experimentation, 24-25, 47, 207

F
Family Planning (*see* Contraception)
Female concerns, 196-197, 207-208
    in correction facilities, 196-197

G
Gay adolescents, 159
Gender identity, 194, 227-229
Groups
    peer pressure, 48, 139-153, 228-229, 170
        for homosexual activity, 156
    use of, 145-152

in skill building, 146-147
in support groups, 147-149
in treatment groups, 149-152
Heterosexual behavior, 92-94, 171, 173-174, 208, 217-218, 233
Historical perspective, 3-16
Homosexual behavior, 25-26, 52-53, 154-166, 171-172, 192-193, 196, 208, 218, 233
  clinical approaches, 159-160
  dealing with, 163-164
  domination and, 54, 157
  experimentation, 25
  gender stress and, 157
  identity confusion and, 157
  institutional adaptation to, 155
  labeling, 161
  peer pressure for, 156
  policy issues regarding, 165-166
  public reaction to, 155
  of staff, 38
  staff attitudes toward, 164-165
  staff-resident behavior, 158
Homosocial environment, 31

I
Identity, 194, 227-229
  development of, 160, 162
Inappropriate sexual behavior, 208
Intimacy
  development of, 40
  in correctional institutions, 196
  need for, 26, 58

K
Kissing and petting, 51, 93

L
Labeling, 161
Language, 99, 106
Legal issues, 51-55, 100
Louis XIII, King
  and masturbation, 4

M
Masturbation, 4, 5, 10-13, 46, 47, 52, 67, 93, 124, 170, 216-217
Mentally handicapped, institutions for, 210-222
  contraception in, 219
  heterosexual behavior in, 217-218
  homosexual behavior in, 218
  masturbation in, 216-217
  normalization in, 211-212
  policies in, 216
  staff attitudes in, 215
  sterilization in, 218
Moral issues, 27-35

N
Neglected and dependent, institutions for, 167-179
Nose-blowing, 6
Normalization, 211-212

O
Organizational structure, in correctional facilities, 198

P
Parent involvement, 23, 39, 67
Peer group influence, 48, 139-153, 228-229, 170
Physically handicapped, institutions for policy in, 22
PLISSIT model of counseling, 110-116
  information giving, 114-115
  permission giving, 113-114
  suggestions, 115-116
Pregnancy, 17, 93 (see also Contraception)
Privacy, 25, 30-31, 45-46, 53, 98-99, 234

R
Rape laws, statutory, 95
Rejection, dealing with, 43
Rights of adolescents in institutions, 21, 24, 33

S
Segregation of the sexes, 28-30, 43-44, 52
Sex education
  of residents, 19-22, 43, 52, 56-70, 178-179
  humor in, 68
  and pregnancy, 44
  and sexually transmitted diseases, 44
  unplanned, 60

Index

of staff, 71-89, 99, 203-205, 232
    and adolescent adjustment, 74
    attitudinal objectives, 86
    common errors, 74
    content of, 84-85
    development of programs, 76
    and expectations of community, 73-74
    and nature of institution, 72-73
    needs determination, 77-78
    objectives of, 80
    and reason for institutionalization, 72
    and social mandates, 73
Sexism
    in correctional facilities, 192
    development of, 31
    and segregation of sexes, 28-30, 43-44, 52
Sexual abuse, 53
Sexual attitudes
    in 17th to 19th centuries, 10-14
    of administration and staff, 29-30
    contemporary, 17-26
    of society, 51, 90-91
    of staff, 17-18, 33-35, 38
Sexual behavior
    heterosexual, 92-94, 171, 173-174, 208, 217-218, 233
    homosexual, 25-26, 52-53, 154-166, 171-172, 192-193, 196, 208, 218, 233
    regulation of, 24
Sexual contact, staff-resident, 90-103
Sexual experimentation, 24-25, 47, 207
Sexual health care, 22-24
Sexual identity, 194, 227-229
    development of, 160-162
Sexual needs, 142-145
Sexual problems and ignorance, 47

Sexually transmitted diseases, 17
Sexuality, control of
    contemporary, 17-26, 51
    17th-19th century, 3-15
Social change, 21
Staff
    resident perceptions of, 172-173
    sexual attitudes of, 17-18, 33-35, 38
    as sexual beings, 96
    sexual contact with residents, 97-101
    as trainers, 18
Staff-resident sexual contact, 97-101
Sterilization of mentally handicapped, 218-219

T

Theraputic intervention (*see also* Counseling), 118-137
    behavioral change procedures, 125-126
    in correction facilities, 194-199
    for decreasing undesired sexual behaviors, 129-132
    evaluation of, 133-134
    for exposing genitals in public, 124
    for inadequate heterosexual skills, 124
    for increasing adaptive sex responses, 127-129
    for indiscriminate choice of partners, 123
    for masturbation in public, 124
    strategies, overview of, 126-127
    therapeutic values, 132-133
    types of problems, 122-123
Touching, staff-resident, 95

V

Values, 37, 39, 132-133
    Conflicts between parents and staff, 39
    of therapeutic interventions, 132-133

ABOUT THE EDITORS

David A. Shore, M.S.W. is program manager for quality assurance in psychiatry and substance abuse for the Joint Commission on Accreditation of Hospitals. He is former director of a private child welfare agency in Chicago. Certified by the American Association of Sex Educators, Counselors, and Therapists in all three categories. Mr. Shore is founding editor of the *Journal of Social Work & Human Sexuality,* editor of the journal *Human Sexuality Update* and is also on the editorial of numerous professional journals. Mr. Shore served on the international scientific committee of the 5th World Congress of Sexology and was chairperson for the Congress symposium, *Sex in Institutions: A Multidimensional Problem.* His text, *Social Work Perspectives in Child Sexual Abuse* will be released shortly.

Harvey L. Gochros, D.S.W. is Professor of Social Work and Director of the Social Work Program for the Study of Sex at the University of Hawaii at Manoa. He is the author of four previous books on sexuality and behavior and numerous articles on social work education and practice with sex-related problems. Professor Gochros has presented many university workshops on social work practice with sexual difficulties. He is also editorial advisor to *Journal of Social Work and Human Sexuality.*

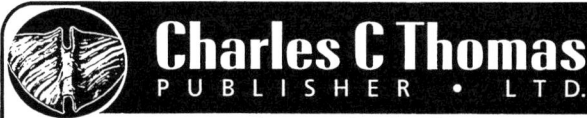

Charles C Thomas
PUBLISHER • LTD.
Leader In Behavioral Sciences Publications

▶ denotes new publication

▶ Landy, Robert J.—**HOW WE SEE GOD AND WHY IT MATTERS: A Multicultural View Through Children's Drawings and Stories.** '01, 230 pp. (8 x 1/2 x 11), 55 il. (40 in color).

▶ Baratta, Larry G.—**A COMPENDIUM OF DEGENERATIVE BRAIN DISEASES: With Sections on Neurophysiology and Neuropharmacology.** '01, 116 pp. (6 x 9), 16 il., paper.

▶ Aiken, Lewis R.—**PERSONALITY: Theories, Assessment, Research, and Applications.** '00, 476 pp. (7 x 10), 24 il., 23 tables, $89.95, cloth, $64.95, paper.

▶ Moser, Rosemarie Scolaro & Corinne E. Frantz—**SHOCKING VIOLENCE: Youth Perpetrators and Victims—A Multidisciplinary Perspective.** '00, 230 pp. (7 x 10), 1 il., 2 tables, $50.95, hard, $33.95, paper.

▶ Sapp, Marty—**HYPNOSIS, DISSOCIATION, AND ABSORPTION: Theories, Assessment and Treatment** '00, 182 pp. (6 x 9), 4 tables, $35.95, cloth, $23.95, paper.

▶ Sumerall, Scott W., Shane J. Lopez and Mary E. Oehlert—**COMPETENCY-BASED EDUCATION AND TRAINING IN PSYCHOLOGY: A Primer.** '00, 130 pp. (6 1/2 x 9 1/2), 1 il., 12 tables, $19.95, paper.

▶ Violanti, John M., Douglas Paton & Christine Dunning—**POSTTRAUMATIC STRESS INTERVENTION: Challenges, Issues, and Perspectives.** '00, 244 pp. (7 x 10), 4 il., 8 tables, $44.95, hard, $31.95, paper.

Dennison, Susan T. & Connie M. Knight—**ACTIVITIES FOR CHILDREN IN THERAPY: A Guide for Planning and Facilitating Therapy with Troubled Children. (2nd Ed.)** '99, 302 pp. (8 1/2 x 11), 201 il., 12 tables, $47.95, spiral (paper).

Bellini, James L. & Phillip D. Rumrill, Jr.—**RESEARCH IN REHABILITATION COUNSELING: A Guide to Design, Methodology, and Utilization.** '99, 252 pp. (7 x 10), 5 tables, $47.95, cloth, $34.95, paper.

Dixon, Charlotte G. & William G. Emener— **PROFESSIONAL COUNSELING: Transitioning into the Next Millennium.** '99, 194 pp. (7 x 10), 2 il., 1 table, $38.95, cloth, $25.95, paper.

Parker, Woodrow M.—**CONSCIOUSNESS-RAISING: A Primer for Multicultural Counseling. (2nd Ed.)** '98, 328 pp. (7 x 10), 2 il., 3 tables, $65.95, cloth, $49.95, paper.

Slovenko, Ralph—**PSYCHOTHERAPY AND CONFIDENTIALITY: Testimonial Privileged Communication, Breach of Confidentiality, and Reporting Duties.** '98, 660 pp. (6 3/4 x 9 3/4), 17 il., $83.95, cloth.

Weikel, William J. & Artis J. Palmo—**FOUNDATIONS OF MENTAL HEALTH COUNSELING. (2nd Ed.)** '96, 446 pp. (7 x 10), 7 il., 1 table, $93.95, cloth, $71.95, paper.

▶ Klausmeier Herbert J.—**RESEARCH WRITING IN EDUCATION AND PSYCHOLOGY—FROM PLANNING TO PUBLICATION: A PRACTICAL HANDBOOK.** '01, 164 pp. (7 x 10).

▶ Fredericks, Lillian E.—**THE USE OF HYPNOSIS IN SURGERY AND ANESTHESIOLOGY: Psychological Preparation of the Surgical Patient.** '00, 280 pp. (7 x 10), 1 il., 3 tables.

▶ Lenchitz, Kenneth—**AUTISM AND POST-TRAUMATIC STRESS DISORDER: Ending Autistic Fixation.** '00, 136 pp. (6 x 9), $36.95, cloth, $19.95, paper.

▶ Lester, David—**WHY PEOPLE KILL THEMSELVES: A 2000 Summary of Research on Suicide. (4th Ed.)** '00, 410 pp. (7 x 10), $89.95, cloth, $62.95, paper.

▶ Thomas, R. Murray—**MULTICULTURAL COUNSELING AND HUMAN DEVELOPMENT THEORIES: 25 Theoretical Perspectives.** '00, 252 pp. (6 1/4 x 9 1/4), $39.95, hard, $26.95, paper.

▶ Thorson, James A.—**PERSPECTIVES ON SPIRITUAL WELL-BEING AND AGING.** '00, 230 pp. (7 x 10), $45.95, cloth, $31.95, paper.

▶ Kendler, Howard H.—**AMORAL THOUGHTS ABOUT MORALITY: The Intersection of Science, Psychology, and Ethics.** '00, 210 pp. (7 x 10), $42.95, cloth, $29.95, paper.

Boy, Angelo V. & Gerald J. Pine—**A PERSON-CENTERED FOUNDATION FOR COUNSELING AND PSYCHOTHERAPY. (2nd Ed.)** '99, 274 pp. (7 x 10), 1 il., 1 table, $57.95, cloth, $41.95, paper.

Taub, Sheila—**RECOVERED MEMORIES OF CHILD SEXUAL ABUSE: Psychological, Social, and Legal Perspectives on a Contemporary Mental Health Controversy.** '99, 234 pp. (7 x 10), 10 il., 4 tables, $46.95, cloth, $33.95, paper.

Jordan, Thomas—**INDIVIDUATION IN CONTEMPORARY PSYCHOANALYSIS. The Emergence of Individuality in Interpersonal and Relational Theory and Practice.** '99, 314 pp. (7 x 10), 1 il., $57.95, cloth, $41.95, paper.

Berger, LeslieBeth—**INCEST, WORK AND WOMEN: Understanding the Consequences of Incest on Women's Careers, Work and Dreams.** '98, 234 pp. (7 x 10), 3 tables, $51.95, cloth, $37.95, paper.

Rugel, Robert P.—**DEALING WITH THE PROBLEM OF LOW SELF-ESTEEM: Common Characteristics and Treatment in Individual, Marital/Family and Group Psychotherapy.** '95, 228 pp. (7 x 10), 2 tables, $50.95, cloth, $37.95, paper.

Ponterotto, Joseph G. & J. Manuel Casas—**HANDBOOK OF RACIAL/ETHNIC MINORITY COUNSELING RESEARCH.** '91, 208 pp. (7 x 10), 18 tables, $43.95, cloth, $31.95, paper.

Books sent on approval • Shipping charges: $5.95 U.S. / $6.95 Canada • Prices subject to change without notice

Contact us to order books or a free catalog with over 800 titles
Call 1-800-258-8980 or 1-217-789-8980 or Fax 1-217-789-9080
2600 South First Street • Springfield • Illinois • 62704
Complete catalog available at www.ccthomas.com • books@ccthomas.com